Language Understanding
Current Issues

SECOND EDITION

27.=

12/28/04			
5-18-12			

Open Guides to Psychology

Series Editor: Judith Greene, Professor of Psychology
at the Open University

Titles in the series

Learning to Use Statistical Tests in Psychology
Judith Greene and Manuela D'Oliveira

Basic Cognitive Processes
Judith Greene and Carolyn Hicks

Memory: Current Issues (Second Edition)
Gillian Cohen, George Kiss and Martin Le Voi

Language Understanding: Current Issues (Second Edition)
Judith Greene and Mark Coulson

Problem Solving: Current Issues (Second Edition)
Hank Kahney

Perception and Representation: Current Issues (Second Edition)
Ilona Roth and Vicki Bruce

Designing and Reporting Experiments
Peter Harris

Biological Foundations of Behaviour
Frederick Toates

Running Applied Psychology Experiments
John Leach

Language Understanding
Current Issues

SECOND EDITION

Parts I and II
by Judith Greene

Part III
by Mark Coulson

Open University Press
Buckingham · Philadelphia

Open University Press
Celtic Court
22 Ballmoor
Buckingham
MK18 1XW

and
1900 Frost Road, Suite 101
Bristol, PA 19007, USA

In association with The Open University

First published 1986 as *Language Understanding: A Cognitive Approach*
Second edition first published 1995

ISBN 0 335 19437 0

A CIP catalogue record for this book is available from the British
Library

Library of Congress Cataloging-in-Publication Data

Greene, Judith.
    Language understanding : current issues / Judith Greene, Mark
Coulson. — 2nd ed.
        p.   cm. — (Open guides to psychology)
    Includes bibliographical references and index.
    ISBN 0–335–19437–0 (pbk.)
    1. Psycholinguistics.   2. Cognition.   3. Competence and
performance (Linguistics)   I. Coulson, Mark, 1956–   . II. Title.
III. Series.
BF455.G737   1995   94–24072
401′.9—dc20   CIP

Edited and designed by The Open University
Typeset by Graphicraft Typesetters Limited, Hong Kong
Printed in Great Britain by Biddles Limited, Guildford and Kings Lynn

(Parts I and II)
To Pat and Julie

(Part III)
Once again, for Ana. The pun is no better now than it was then

Language Understanding

Contents

Preface	11
Acknowledgements	11
Introduction	13
How to use this guide	14
Part I Language and Knowledge	15
Judith Greene	
1 Introduction	17
1.1 Definitions of language	17
1.2 Competence and performance	17
1.3 Lexical meanings and syntax	19
1.4 Semantics and general knowledge	20
1.5 Language in context	21
2 The lexicon	23
2.1 Word meanings	23
2.2 Semantic features	25
2.3 Semantic cases	25
2.4 Semantic primitives	26
3 Syntactic structures	27
3.1 Chomsky's theory of syntactic competence	27
3.2 The structure of linguistic competence	31
3.3 Psychological tests of Chomsky's linguistic theory	32
4 Semantic representations	34
4.1 Semantic features and semantic representations	35
4.2 Case frames and semantic representations	36
4.3 Semantic primitives and semantic representations	37
4.4 Syntax or semantics?	38
5 Representations of discourse	40
5.1 Story grammars	40
5.2 Representations of events as scripts	42

5.3	Representations of texts as macrostructures	44
5.4	The effort after meaning: making inferences	45
6	**Some conclusions**	47
Further reading		49

Part II Language Processes and Models 51
Judith Greene

1	**Introduction**	53
1.1	Modular models	54
1.2	A linear model	54
1.3	An interactive model	55
1.4	Methods of investigation	57
2	**Lexical processing and semantic processing**	58
2.1	Semantic priming experiments	59
2.2	Cross-modal semantic priming experiments	60
2.3	The role of the lexicon in computer models	65
2.4	Cottrell's lexically-based model	67
3	**Syntactic processing and semantic processing**	69
3.1	Grammatical judgements	70
3.2	Effects of syntactic priming	70
3.3	The role of syntactic parsers in computer models	73
3.4	Winograd's interactive model of language understanding	78
4	**Discourse processing and general knowledge**	81
4.1	General knowledge inferences: scripts revisited	82
4.2	St John's story gestalt model	83
5	**Concluding issues**	87
Further reading		89

Part III Anaphoric Reference 91
Mark Coulson

1	**Introduction**	93
1.1	What is anaphoric reference?	93
1.2	Why study anaphors?	93
1.3	Some terminology	97
2	**Types of anaphor**	98
2.1	Pro-anaphors	99
2.2	Noun phrase anaphors	100

2.3	Ellipsis	101
2.4	Deixis, sense and reference	103
3	**Processing anaphors**	105
3.1	Two models of anaphoric processing	105
3.2	The time-course of information use	107
3.3	Finding antecedents: the rules of resolution	110
3.4	Lexical information and non-linguistic information	113
3.5	Breaking the rules	116
3.6	Returning to the models	118
4	**Placing anaphors in context**	119
4.1	Focus	119
4.2	Sentential focus	121
4.3	Discourse focus	123
4.4	Anaphor antecedent distance	127
4.5	Intonation	129
5	**The bonding process**	131
5.1	The final interpretation	131
5.2	The immediacy of resolution and anaphoric ambiguity	132
5.3	Anaphors and inferences	135
6	**Conclusions**	136

Overview

139

Judith Greene

Answers to SAQs	143
References	149
Index of Authors	153
Index of Concepts	155

Preface

Within the Open Guides to Psychology series, *Language Understanding* is one of a companion set of four books, the others being *Memory, Problem Solving* and *Perception and Representation*. Together these form the main texts of the Open University third-level course in Cognitive Psychology, but each of the four volumes can be read independently. The course is designed for second or third year students. It is presented in the style and format that the Open University has found to be uniquely effective in making the material intelligible and interesting.

The books provide an up-to-date, in-depth treatment of some of the major issues, theories and findings in cognitive psychology. They are designed to introduce a representative selection of different research methods, and the reader is encouraged, by means of Activities and Self-assessment Questions interpolated through the text, to become involved in cognitive psychology as an active participant.

The authors gratefully acknowledge the many helpful comments and suggestions of fellow members of the course team and of the external assessor Michael W. Eysenck on earlier drafts, and the valuable assistance of Pat Vasiliou in typing the manuscript.

Acknowledgements

Grateful acknowledgement is made to the following sources for permission to reproduce material in this book:

Figure 1.9: adapted from Bower, G.H., Black, J.B. and Turner, T.J. (1979) 'Scripts in text comprehension and memory', *Cognitive Psychology*, 11, pp.177–220, Academic Press Inc.; *Figure 2.3:* adapted from Cottrell, G.W. (1989) *A Connectionist Approach to Word Sense Disambiguation*, Pitman Publishers; *Figure 2.5:* adapted from Winograd, T. (1972) *Understanding Natural Language*, Academic Press Inc.; *Figure 2.7:* adapted from St John, M.F. (1992) 'The story gestalt: a model of knowledge-intensive processes in text comprehension', *Cognitive Science*, 16, pp. 271–306, Ablex Publishing Corporation.

Introduction

This book is divided into three parts, each of which introduces a different approach to language understanding. Part I emphasizes the enormous amount of knowledge required to explain our ability to understand what we hear and read. To start with, we have to know the vocabulary and grammar of a language. But, as you have probably realized if you have ever tried to learn a foreign language, much more is required in order to be able to communicate effectively. Apart from many idiomatic phrases, a speaker has to know the social conventions for language use. Finally, if you know nothing about the topic under discussion, you are not likely to understand much about what is being said.

Part II focuses on the various types of processes which underlie language use. These include accessing word definitions, applying grammatical rules and the processes involved in understanding a whole text, story or newspaper article. One issue which emerges is whether different sources of knowledge interact in language processing. In building up interpretations of words and sentences and whole texts, at what point do we bring to bear all the different sorts of expectations which determine how we are likely to interpret language?

Part III addresses these same issues in the area of anaphoric reference. This term is used to describe the processes by which language users understand the links between pronouns and other words in a sentence. Are these due to purely linguistic processes, such as knowing that *she* must refer to a female? Or is it necessary to bring in knowledge about the situations being described in order to identify which woman is being referred to?

The relation between the specifically linguistic knowledge which is necessary to speak a language and more general knowledge is a constant theme throughout this book. Experiments which tap language processes and conclusions drawn from attempts to produce computer programs which simulate human language understanding have produced fascinating and sometimes contradictory evidence about the processes underlying language understanding. The Overview at the end of the book provides a commentary highlighting the many problematic issues involved in studying language.

Perhaps we should end this introduction by stating which areas of language understanding will not be covered in this book. There will be nothing about how speech sounds are analysed or how individual letters are recognized as words. Important as these problems are for theories of speech perception and reading, they would require another book to deal with them adequately. In this volume, the language understanding process is taken as starting at the point when language users have recognized spoken or written words. The problem of how they attribute meanings to individual words, sentences and texts raises complex issues which are of special relevance to cognitive psychology.

How to use this guide

In each section of this book you will find Self-Assessment Questions (SAQs) inserted at various points in the text. Attempting all the SAQs should give you a better understanding of theoretical issues and research techniques. They will also help to make you an active participant instead of just a passive reader. The answers can be found at the end of the book and will help to illuminate points made in the text.

Detailed accounts of experiments are presented in Techniques Boxes; these are chosen to illustrate commonly used experimental methods. The Summaries at the end of each section recapitulate the main points and so provide a useful aid to revision. The Index of Concepts that appears at the end of the book indicates the place in the text where each concept is first introduced and defined. Entries in the Index of Concepts are emboldened in the text.

Part I
Language and Knowledge

Judith Greene

Part I Language and Knowledge

Contents

1   Introduction   17
1.1   Definitions of language   17
1.2   Competence and performance   17
1.3   Lexical meanings and syntax   19
1.4   Semantics and general knowledge   20
1.5   Language in context   21

2   The lexicon   23
2.1   Word meanings   23
2.2   Semantic features   25
2.3   Semantic cases   25
2.4   Semantic primitives   26

3   Syntactic structures   27
3.1   Chomsky's theory of syntactic competence   27
3.2   The structure of linguistic competence   31
3.3   Psychological tests of Chomsky's linguistic theory   32

4   Semantic representations   34
4.1   Semantic features and semantic representations   35
4.2   Case frames and semantic representations   36
4.3   Semantic primitives and semantic representations   37
4.4   Syntax or semantics?   38

5   Representations of discourse   40
5.1   Story grammars   40
5.2   Representations of events as scripts   42
5.3   Representations of texts as macrostructures   44
5.4   The effort after meaning: making inferences   45

6   Some conclusions   47

Further reading   49

1   Introduction

Conventionally, language is defined as having two main functions: external communications with other people and internal representations of our own thoughts. The advent of writing has resulted in so many written records that years of education are now deemed necessary for children to learn the accumulated history and scientific discoveries of their culture — the 'thinking' of past generations. It is difficult to conceive how any civilization could exist without developing some method for communicating thoughts.

In the light of this, it may seem a trivial matter to define language and communication. You may be surprised to hear that whole books have been written to try to answer the questions 'what is language?' and 'what is communication?'

1.1   Definitions of language

The problem is that these terms can be used in so many ways. 'Language is unique to human beings' refers to language as an ability which is universal to all humans and only humans. 'English is a rich and flexible language' refers to one of the many human languages, the one which happens to be spoken by members of English-speaking societies and by many other people as a second language. 'The English language is derived from Latin and Anglo-Saxon roots': this suggests that a language 'exists' as an entity in its own right with a history of change over the centuries. 'John knows English' refers to language as part of an individual's knowledge. 'John speaks English well' implies that there can be variations in the way individuals use a generally accepted language. 'John said he was going home' is a particular utterance which can be understood by any speaker of the English language. 'John's home is over there' is an utterance which will only communicate something in a context in which it is obvious what 'over there' means. 'It's chilly' can be interpreted as a comment about the weather or as a request to close the window. A shrug of the shoulders may communicate disinterest.

1.2   Competence and performance

I am certainly not going to try to sort out all the terminological issues which have puzzled philosophers and linguists for hundreds of years. There is, however, one important distinction you should bear in mind. This is a contrast which has often been made between competence and

17

performance. **Competence** refers to people's knowledge of a language, the knowledge that enables them to produce and understand utterances in that language. **Performance** refers to the actual production and comprehension of utterances, whether in speech or writing. Any faults or hesitations in speech or writing are thought to be due to temporary lapses which affect performance but do not necessarily reflect on people's underlying competence.

The idea behind this distinction is that people 'know' the vocabulary and grammatical rules of any language they can speak. This represents their competence in that language. In performance, speakers may hesitate, make grammatical errors or repeat themselves; listeners may misinterpret what is said to them. Competence is sometimes described as a speaker's 'ideal' knowledge of language. This is contrasted with performance factors, such as forgetting what you meant to say, and relying on non-linguistic cues to make the speaker's meaning clear, which may affect the production and comprehension of individual utterances.

The competence–performance distinction arose out of the discipline of linguistics. **Linguistics** is the study of languages as linguistic systems. Linguists describe the phonetic sound patterns, grammars and vocabularies of languages. (In this context linguists are academics who study linguistics — not necessarily fluent speakers of several languages.) It was a well-known linguist Noam Chomsky (1965) who crystallized the competence–performance distinction. Modern linguists claim to be describing the competence underlying normal language usage, rather than prescribing what constitutes 'good grammar'. Nevertheless, they are looking for grammatical rules which will explain our ability to recognize and produce correct sentences (i.e. linguistic competence). From this point of view, slips of the tongue or spelling errors can be considered irrelevant, if not positively misleading.

A diametrically opposed view is that it is language use which is all important. Psychologists are naturally interested in the performance factors which affect the way people actually use language. Even within linguistics there are researchers known as **sociolinguists** because of their interest in the social functions of language. They observe how people tailor their speech, and use non-verbal signals to convey meanings appropriate to the social situation and the social status of the speakers and listeners.

Cognitive psychology sits somewhat uneasily between those two extremes. Cognitive psychologists are concerned with mental representations; so they, like the linguists, are interested in how the knowledge underlying language use is represented in the mind. They are equally committed to investigating the mental processes which are responsible for the production and understanding of individual utterances appropriate to the context in which they occur.

Part I of this book will be mainly concerned with the representations of linguistic and other types of knowledge which constitute the competence of the language user who knows a particular language. In *Part II* the processes underlying language performance will be explored.

So the next thing to consider is how we go about finding out what kind of knowledge representations are needed to account for linguistic competence in a particular language.

Just to convince you that there is something here which needs explaining, consider an imaginary tribe called the Shivasi, who live in the desert, hoard every drop of water and worship water spirits. Can you understand the following sentence in the Shivasi language? *Psiht Shivasi gor brok me Babwe fyp.* No, of course you can't. But all members of the Shivasi tribe can! So what does one need to know about a language in order to understand it?

1.3 *Lexical meanings and syntax*

Sometimes the writing system of a language may be unfamiliar: for instance, the text might be in Russian, Persian or Hebrew script. Luckily the Shivasi language uses 'English' letters. So the first thing you might want to ask is what each of the individual words means. Suppose I tell you that in Shivasi *psiht* means 'look'; *Shivasi* means 'Shivasi'; *gor* means 'water'; *brok* means 'then'; *me* means 'not'; *Babwe* means 'Babwe'; *fyp* means 'run'. Are you any the wiser about what *Look Shivasi water then not Babwe run* means? The meanings of words are termed **lexical meanings** (from **lexicon** which is another word for a dictionary). What is obvious from the above example is that knowing the lexical meanings of words is not sufficient to elucidate the meaning of a whole utterance. The next question to consider is how individual words are combined into meaningful utterances. **Syntax** is the technical term for what you probably think of as the grammar of a language. Syntax includes rules for combining words in certain orders and adding appropriate **inflections** (i.e. adding endings to words such as *ed* to indicate the past tense, or *s* to form plurals).

It may seem quite a simple matter to formulate the syntactic rules for a language. But imagine trying to explain to a foreigner why it is possible to say, *Are you coming or aren't you?* but not *Am I coming or amp't I?* Why is it grammatical to say *He walked in* but not *He camed in*; or *two houses* but not *two mouses*? And, of course, there are hundreds of similar cases. If you have ever tried to explain examples like these, you will appreciate the task of a linguist attempting to formalize all the rules which are required to produce grammatically correct English sentences.

In the Shivasi sentence you would have to know that the form of the word *Shivasi* indicates that it is the subject of the sentence. Used as an adjective in the phrase *a Shivasi tent* the word would have a different ending, *Shivasia*. You would also have to know that the first and last words of a Shivasi sentence always make up the main verb; also that *then not* refers to the present time because the Shivasi language always refers to the past unless it is specifically denied. So now you know that the sentence has the following grammatical structure: *Shivasi* (subject) *look/run* (main verb) *then not* (present tense) *water Babwe*. But you may still be puzzled about what the sentence really means.

1.4   Semantics and general knowledge

All members of the Shivasi tribe know that *Babwe* is the name of a forest; and that *look run water* means 'explore' (because of their obsession about water!). And there is no need to specify how many Shivasi there are because they never go exploring except in a group of at least thirty people. So a fluent speaker of Shivasi would immediately understand that the sentence means 'At least thirty of my people are at present exploring the Babwe forest'. The analysis of the meanings of utterances is known as **semantics** (semantics is simply another term for study of meanings).

You may be thinking that the Shivasi sentence is an exaggerated example. But what would a Shivasi make of the English sentence: *Visiting aunts can be a nuisance*?

SAQ 1
(a) Did you notice that the 'aunts' sentence has two quite different meanings?
(b) If the Shivasi had a custom which forbade young girls to visit older female relatives, which meaning would be likely to be selected?
(c) What if older female relatives always had to stay at home?

These examples demonstrate the importance of knowledge about social contexts in determining the meanings of utterances. Indeed, one problem is that the general knowledge needed to interpret the meanings of utterances is potentially unlimited. The two meanings of the sentence *Visiting aunts can be a nuisance* may be semantically comprehensible to any English speaker. However, in a society in which aunts were always respected and loved, neither meaning of the 'visiting aunts' sentence would be acceptable as a communicative statement.

A visiting linguist might learn from his investigations of the Shivasi language that *Shivasi* is the plural form of a noun, but he would need to be an anthropologist to discover that the Shivasi never go exploring except in groups of thirty. When I saw on a poster 'THE POLICE

LIVE AT THE ALBERT HALL', how did I understand this to mean that a pop group, famous at the time, would be performing in person, rather than that members of the constabulary inhabited that vast building? The point about these examples is that they raise the issue of whether all our 'real-life' knowledge about aunts and what goes on at the Albert Hall should be included in our linguistic knowledge of the English language. The relationship between purely linguistic knowledge of a language and general knowledge about the world remains one of the most problematic issues in cognitive theories of language.

1.5   Language in context

So far we have been talking as if meanings can be allocated to individual sentences regardless of the linguistic context in which they are used. But the Shivasi sentence might have been part of a long story about the Shivasi exploring the forest in search of a lost girl. This would set up expectations about how succeeding sentences should be interpreted (e.g. *She had wandered far*). Analysis of the **linguistic context** in which a sentence is embedded is called **discourse analysis**. Discourse refers to the text or conversation in which a sentence is embedded.

Sentences in isolation are often ambiguous and require a linguistic context to disambiguate them. Even a very simple sentence like *He gave her a ring* may be given a different interpretation depending on whether it occurs in the linguistic context of *John asked Mary to marry him* or *John wanted to talk to Mary*. There are many other utterances which only make sense if both participants are aware of the same situation. For example, *Put it next to the big one* can only be understood if the listener can see the objects being discussed; this is sometimes termed **situational context.**

Finally, there is the use of language in a **social context**. When people use language in a face-to-face situation they are usually trying to achieve some aim, such as persuading, showing off, or requesting information. This level of analysis is sometimes called **pragmatic** because it takes into account the purpose of language in achieving pragmatic ends. The use of language to perform particular functions has also been analysed as **speech acts** (Searle, 1970). The speech act of 'requesting' (e.g. to get someone to close a window) may be expressed as a question (*Will you close the window?*), a statement (*It's chilly in here*) or as a direct command (*Close that window*). The way people interpret these utterances depends on their appreciation of a speaker's intentions.

To end with an example from our — totally imaginary — Shivasi tribe, a speaker might have chosen a slightly different phraseology to refer to the exploration of the Babwe forest depending on whether it was in reply to a query from his chief about how many people were left in the village to take part in a ceremony, as opposed to telling a close friend it was too late for him to join the exploring party.

Most examples of language use involve some form of interaction, either face-to-face or between writers and readers. Utterances are never produced in a vacuum but are embedded in a linguistic, situational or social context.

From what I have said so far it is obvious that, as language speakers, we must have competence in the vocabulary and syntax of our language. In addition, we need to know a lot about the world and the conventions for acceptable communications in our society. Without this, we may be able to produce correct grammatical sentences but fail to communicate what we mean to other speakers or to the readers of our written communications.

For cognitive psychologists, these issues can be rephrased as asking how such knowledge is represented in memory. Is our knowledge of grammatical rules represented as a special syntactic component in memory? Is our dictionary of lexical meanings separate from our general knowledge of the world to which they refer? Do we, for instance, store the meaning of the word 'tree' as a tall plant separately from our general knowledge about trees? How is our knowledge about social conventions organized so as to constrain our utterances to make sense?

What we are really talking about here is the whole of human memory. In order to narrow down the problem to manageable proportions, the linguistic knowledge required for language use has been broken down into several topics which have tended to be studied in isolation from each other. In the remaining sections of Part I we shall consider the different types of knowledge representations required to use and understand a language.

Summary of Section 1

- Traditionally, the types of knowledge required for language understanding have been divided into the following categories:
  - (a) Lexical meanings: meanings of words listed in a lexicon (dictionary).
  - (b) Syntax: grammatical rules for combining words in sentences, including word order and word endings (inflections).
  - (c) Semantics: rules for combining word meanings into meaningful sentences.

(d) Discourse analysis: analysis of linguistic context.
(e) Pragmatics: the use of language to communicate intentions by speech acts in social contexts.

2   The lexicon

Most theories of language agree that language users must have some sort of **lexicon** stored in memory. When we hear or read words, it is assumed that the patterns of sounds or letters are recognized because they correspond to a **lexical item** in our mental lexicons. But what are these lexical items like and how do they represent the meanings of words? It may at first appear as if this is an easy question, but in fact most words in a language's vocabulary have many different meanings.

2.1   Word meanings

The ability to recognize words is not a simple perceptual skill, since words are made up of arbitrary sequences of sounds and letters. For instance, English speakers can recognize and pronounce the word *tree* whereas French speakers can recognize and pronounce the word *arbre*, the French word for tree. As you will certainly appreciate if you have tried to learn the vocabulary of a foreign language, it is no easy task to learn the connections between words and their meanings. Moreover, word meanings not only determine how words should be used but often affect the way they should be pronounced. The word *bank* is easy enough to pronounce, although it may have several meanings. But what about *sow*? Should it rhyme with low or cow? This clearly depends on which meaning of the three letters *s-o-w* is intended.

SAQ 2
(a) Write down two sentences, one of which might lead someone to pronounce *bow* to rhyme with *low* and the other to rhyme with *bough*.
(b) Write down at least three meanings for the word *bank*.

The vocabulary problem is highlighted by the fact that in French the word *banque* refers only to a financial institution. The French word for a river bank is *rive*, which can also be used to refer to a beach or coastline. Trying to specify all the possible senses of words, as in a dictionary, is a never-ending task. It was only when I was looking up the word for river bank in my French dictionary that I noticed that *rivière de diamants* means a diamond necklace, an enchanting phrase although 'river of diamonds' would have quite a different sense in English. The problem is, if words can have so many different meanings, how do we know which sense is intended? If the word *bank* is so ambiguous, how do we know whether it means a financial institution or the edge of a river?

While some words are relatively easy to define by pointing to an object or a picture (e.g. *camel, zebra* or *unicorn*), many — perhaps most — depend on the context in which they occur. There is, for instance, unlikely to be much confusion about *I needed some money, so I went to the bank*. A nice demonstration of the importance of context in defining word meanings comes from Schank (1982). Schank chose as an example the way that an apparently simple word like *took* changes its meaning according to the sentence in which it occurs. The primary meaning of *took* might be thought of as implying that one person has taken something away from someone else. But does this cover the meaning of *took* in all the following sentences?

> *John took the book*
> *John took an aeroplane*
> *John took an aspirin*
> *John took the job*
> *John took my advice*
> *Schank took as an example . . .*

All these sentences seem to share a common core of meaning and yet there are subtle distinctions, as shown by the fact that the word *grabbed*, which might be thought of as a synonym for *took*, only sounds right in the first sentence. A **synonym** is a word with an identical or similar meaning.

SAQ 3
Write down an appropriate synonym (either a word or a phrase) for *gave* in each of the following sentences:
(a) *John gave Mary a (wedding) ring.*
(b) *John gave Mary a (telephone) ring.*
(c) *John gave Mary a cold.*
(d) *John gave in.*
(e) *John gave notice.*

Psychological theories of language aim to describe how people know which sense of a word to select in any particular context. Why do language users find no problem in deciding that *the pen in the box* implies quite a different meaning for the word *pen* as compared with *the box in the pen*? Why are we usually quite unaware of the possible ambiguity of the word *ring* in a sentence referring to a ring for your finger or a telephone call?

Sections 2.2 to 2.4 describe three approaches to tackling the problem of representing word meanings in such a way that the correct senses of words can be selected: semantic features, case frames and semantic primitives.

2.2   Semantic features

The basic idea behind this approach is that all the words in the lexicon can be defined in terms of sets of **semantic features**. Katz and Fodor (1963) proposed a theory in which words are defined in terms of features like animate, inanimate, human, animal, physical object, activity. Each sense of a word would have to be allocated different features, as shown for the word *ball* in Figure 1.1.

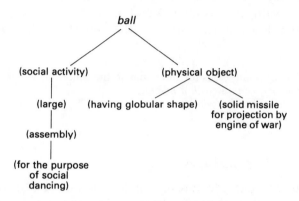

Figure 1.1   Semantic features (adapted from Katz and Fodor, 1963)

Another way of expressing information about semantic features is to list for each sense of a word whether it has a feature (+) or doesn't have it (−). An example would be *ball* (+ physical object) (− human) and *ball* (+ social activity) (+ large) (+ assembly).

SAQ 4
Write down some features (+ and −) for the word *bachelor*.

2.3   Semantic cases

Semantic features represent word meanings in terms of features which define that word. Another quite different approach is to define words in terms of the sentence contexts in which they occur.

One of the most common types of analysis of sentence contexts is known as **case grammar**. First proposed by the linguist Fillmore (1968), the basic idea is to represent verbs in terms of 'cases' attached to the verb. The main cases are listed below:

Agent: animate being who initiates action
Instrument: inanimate entity which is involved in the action
Recipient: animate being who is affected by the action
Object: inanimate entity which is affected by the action
Locative: the location or direction of the action

The Object is defined as any inanimate entity which is affected by the verb, whether or not it is the grammatical object of the verb. For instance, in *The picture was painted by John*, the *picture* would be the Object because it is affected by being painted by John (the Agent). In a sentence like *The key opened the door*, the *key* is treated as an Instrument (with an unstated Agent representing the person who unlocked the door) and the *door* as the Object which is affected by 'opening'.

SAQ 5
Indicate the appropriate cases for the nouns in the following sentences:
(a) *John broke the window with a hammer.*
(b) *The hammer broke the window.*
(c) *John invited Mary to a party.*

2.4 Semantic primitives

Rather than attributing features to whole words, some researchers have attempted to capture the semantic core of word meanings by 'decomposing' their meanings into a small set of **semantic primitives**. Schank (1972) drew up a list of 12–15 **primitive actions** which he claims underlie the meanings of all verbs which describe actions. Listed below are some of Schank's main primitives, which he calls **Acts**:

ATRANS: transfer of possession
PTRANS: physical transfer from one location to another
MTRANS: transfer of mental information
MBUILD: build memory structures
ATTEND: sensory input (seeing, hearing, etc.)
PROPEL: application of force to physical object
MOVE: move a body part
INGEST: intake of food, air
EXPEL: the reverse of ingest!

SAQ 6
List the primitive Acts which best express the meanings of the verbs in the following sentences:
(a) *Mary gave John a book.*
(b) *Mary gave John some advice.*

(c) *Mary took a plane.*
(d) *Mary took an aspirin.*
(e) *Mary raised her arm.*
(f) *Mary raised her consciousness.*

According to Schank, for each verb in the lexicon there is a list of the possible primitives it can express. For instance, a word like *give* would be defined as having at least two senses: 'transfer of possession' (ATRANS) and 'transfer of mental information' (MTRANS), as in *Mary gave some advice to John.*

Summary of Section 2

- The lexicon contains representations of word definitions which allow language users to select appropriate senses of words in sentence contexts.
- One way of defining words is in terms of semantic features like (+ physical object) (+ animal) (+ human). These features are used to express differences between permitted and non-permitted combinations of words.
- Another way of defining words is to formulate them as cases (Agent, Object, Instrument, etc.) which particular verbs require.
- A third way is to decompose words into semantic primitives so that the meanings of all verbs which map on to the same primitive action can be analysed in the same way.

3   Syntactic structures

The message of the previous section was that it is not enough to know the meanings of individual words in order to understand sentences. In fact, it is very hard to define the meanings of many commonly used words, like *give* and *take*, without indicating the different meanings they could have in different sentence contexts. So in this section we shall be considering the role of grammatical combinations of words in understanding sentences.

3.1   Chomsky's theory of syntactic competence

Noam Chomsky is a linguist who has had a great influence on theories about the role of syntax in sentence understanding. He argues that our ability to recognize and understand grammatical English sentences is evidence that we must 'know' the rules of English grammar. For instance, anyone who knows English knows that *Colourless green ideas sleep furiously* is a grammatical sentence — although it is nonsense — while *Ideas green furiously colourless sleep* is ungrammatical.

Chomsky's theory is intended to formalize the rules which constitute linguistic competence: in other words, the knowledge which enables language speakers to identify some sequences of words as grammatical and others ungrammatical, as with the 'colourless ideas' example. One important point made by Chomsky is that it is impossible to list all the sentences that might conceivably be spoken in a particular language. The linguistic rules must therefore be capable of generating all possible grammatical sentences in a language whether they have ever been spoken before or not. Because it is a theory about competence, Chomsky's grammar says nothing about the actual processes people use to produce or understand sentences.

Chomsky's linguistic theory was the first to draw psychologists' attention to the syntactic rules of language. Before Chomsky (BC!), psychologists had mainly concentrated on the processing of single words, for the simple reason that they had no method for representing the structure of larger units like sentences and texts. Chomsky's demonstration that people are able to identify the 'grammaticality' of sentences was interpreted as supporting the idea that language involves parsing sentences into grammatical categories.

Chomsky's theory of grammar takes the form of rules for generating sentences. His use of the term *generative rules* has given rise to the mistaken view that Chomsky is postulating the rules language speakers actually use to produce utterances. Since Chomsky's is a competence theory, the term 'generating' is neutral about performance, being concerned only with the grammatical rules which distinguish between grammatical and ungrammatical combinations of words. A simple example of the rules in Chomsky's (1957) grammar is shown in Figure 1.2.

1	S (sentence)	⟶	NP (noun phrase) + VP (verb phrase)
2	NP	⟶	N (noun)
3	NP	⟶	article + N
4	NP	⟶	adjective + N
5	NP	⟶	pronoun
6	VP	⟶	V (verb) + NP
7	VP	⟶	V + adjective
8	N	⟶	*Jane, boy, girl, apples*
9	V	⟶	*likes, hit, was hit, was, are cooking, are*
10	adjective	⟶	*good, unfortunate, cooking*
11	article	⟶	*a, the*
12	pronoun	⟶	*he, she, they*

Figure 1.2 Simplified version of Chomsky's rules

These rules are known as **rewrite rules** because they rewrite a sentence into its constituent parts. According to Rule 1, the symbol for sentence (S) can be rewritten into symbols standing for noun phrase (NP) and verb phrase (VP). What this first rule is really saying is that sentences in English consist of a noun phrase followed by a verb phrase.

Rules 2–5 state that an NP can be rewritten either as an N (noun), e.g. *Jane*; or as an article plus N, e.g. *The boy*; or as an adjective plus N, e.g. *cooking apples*; or as a pronoun, e.g. *he*. Rules 6 and 7 state that a VP can be rewritten as a V (verb) and NP; or as a V and adjective. The NP introduced in Rule 6 can itself be rewritten according to Rules 2–5. Finally, Rules 8–12 allow the symbols to be rewritten as actual words. These rewriting rules can be used to produce *syntactic trees* which define the **syntactic structures** of sentences. An example of the way the rules can be used to generate a syntactic tree structure for a particular sentence is shown in Figure 1.3.

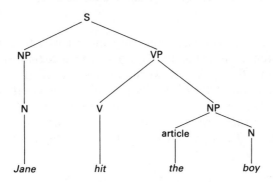

Figure 1.3   Syntactic tree structure

Syntactic tree structures show which of the rules have been used to generate a sentence. The rules keep being applied until all the symbols, e.g. NP, VP, N, V are rewritten as actual words. For instance, the rules used to generate the *Jane hit the boy* tree are rules 1, 2, 6, 3, 8, 9, 11, 8. Make sure that you follow this example through, checking how each rule was used to generate the syntactic tree.

SAQ 7
Using the grammar in Figure 1.2, draw a syntactic tree structure for the sentence *Jane was unfortunate.*

One great advantage of rewrite rules is that they can be used to specify different syntactic structures for sentences which have syntactically ambiguous structures. The sentence *They are cooking apples* can be analysed in two different ways, depending on whether it refers to a particular type of apple (cooking apples) or to the fact that people (they) are cooking (V) apples (see Figure 1.4).

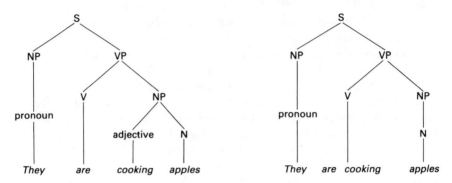

Figure 1.4   Syntactic structures of ambiguous sentence

Chomsky (1957) proposed that the simplest way to generate more complex sentences like passives is to use **transformational rules** for changing round the order of words in a sentence. For instance, an active sentence like *Jane hit the boy* would be generated directly by rewriting rules to generate the tree structure shown in Figure 1.3. This would then be 'transformed' by reordering the words in order to produce the passive *The boy was hit by Jane* (see Figure 1.5).

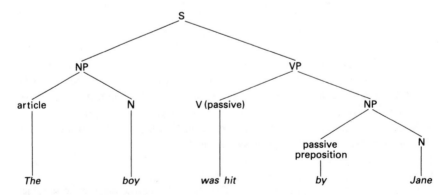

Figure 1.5   Syntactic structure of passive sentence

The passive transformation rule states that, when *Jane hit the boy* is transformed, the passive form of the verb (*was hit*) and the preposition *by* should be selected to produce *The boy was hit by Jane*.

3.2   The structure of linguistic competence

In a later version of his theory, Chomsky (1965) made explicit the notion that each sentence has a **surface structure** and a **deep structure**. The surface structure represents the actual order of the words in a sentence, for instance, *The boy was hit by Jane.* The deep structure represents the basic grammatical relationships from which such a sentence is derived (i.e. *Jane hit the boy*).

SAQ 8
Which pairs of sentences have similar deep structures and which have similar surface structures?
(a) *A new student painted the picture.*
(b) *The picture was painted by a new student.*
(c) *The picture was painted by a new technique.*

Chomsky went on to suggest that deep structures contain all the syntactic information necessary for interpreting the meanings of sentences. Surface structures, on the other hand, are necessary for representing the words of a sentence in the correct order. A complete grammar must specify transformational rules for mapping surface structures on to deep structures and vice versa. Figure 1.6 shows the relationship between deep and surface structures in Chomsky's theory. You should note that there are no arrows shown between the boxes to emphasize that it is a model of linguistic competence which is 'neutral' about how language users actually process linguistic inputs.

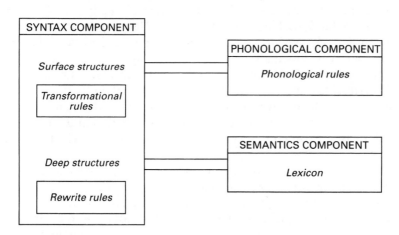

Figure 1.6   Chomsky's (1965) theory of language

The **syntax component** consists of (a) rewrite rules for generating deep structures and (b) transformational rules which map these deep structures on to surface structures. Surface structures feed into the **phonological component** which contains phonological rules for generating the sounds of the words in the correct order. Deep structures provide all the syntactic information necessary for semantic analysis and are fed into the **semantics component**. An essential characteristic of Chomsky's model, as shown in Figure 1.6, is that the components are entirely separate. In particular, it is only after the rules in the syntax component have fully completed the analysis of deep structures that they are input into the semantics component. Chomsky's transformational grammar represents in its most extreme form the claim that syntax and semantics are quite distinct types of analysis.

3.3   Psychological tests of Chomsky's linguistic theory

Chomsky's model gave rise to a lot of psychological research in the 1960s and 1970s. The term **psycholinguistics** was coined to emphasize the marriage between *psychology* and Chomsky's *linguistic* theory. Psycholinguists carried out experiments to test whether people's ability to memorize and evaluate the meanings of sentences is affected by the number and complexity of transformations needed to generate the sentences.

When faced with psychological evidence, Chomsky reiterated that his theory is intended to represent the linguistic competence of language speakers. The evidence relevant to his grammar is whether (a) it accounts for the generation of grammatical sentences, ruling out ungrammatical sentences, and (b) it provides all the information which is necessary for describing the competence of language users. The theory of deep and surface structures (shown in Figure 1.6) does, however, imply that syntactic analysis is a separate stage in linguistics and that semantics does not get involved until a syntactic analysis is completed.

Experiments have been carried out demonstrating that it is unlikely that people perform a transformational syntactic analysis and only then consider a semantic interpretation. A classic experiment demonstrating an interaction between syntax and semantics is described in Techniques Box A.

Slobin interpreted the finding that irreversible passives are relatively easy as demonstrating that the semantic implausibility of flowers watering girls offsets the syntactic complexity of a passive transformation. These findings, and other similar results, cast doubt on the contention that syntactic analysis into deep structures must be completed before the semantics component can start to work. People make assumptions about what a sentence might plausibly mean and, indeed, may sometimes bypass syntactic analysis altogether (e.g. assuming that it must be the girl who is doing the watering).

TECHNIQUES BOX A

Slobin's Sentence Verification Experiment (1966)

Rationale
According to Chomsky's (1957) theory, active sentences (A) require
no transformations, passive sentences (P) require a single passive
transformation to reorder the words, negatives (N) require a single
negative transformation, and passive negative (PN) sentences require
two transformations. It was predicted that subjects would take longer
to evaluate sentences requiring more transformations.

Method
Sentences of various types were presented to subjects (Ss) along with
a picture (see examples below). The sentences had to be judged as
true (T) or false (F) depending on how they described the scene in
the picture, known as a *sentence verification task*.

Sentence	Picture
The girl is watering the flowers (A)	Girl watering flowers (T)
The dog is being chased by the cat (P)	Dog chasing cat (F)
The girl is not watering the flowers (N)	Girl watering flowers (F)
The cat is not being chased by the dog (PN)	Cat chasing dog (T)

Some of the sentences were called 'reversible' because the subject
and object could be reversed and still result in a sensible sentence,
e.g. *The dog is chasing the cat* or *The cat is chasing the dog*. Other
sentences were 'irreversible' because switching the subject and object
resulted in a nonsensical sentence, e.g. *The flowers are watering the girl*.

Results
Reaction times to verify true sentences (seconds):

	A	P	N	PN
Reversible	0.93	1.21	1.27	1.75
Irreversible	0.70	0.69	0.98	1.01

As you can see from the table, in general active (A) sentences were
verified most quickly while passive negative (PN) sentences took the
longest times. However, a surprising finding was that, with the irreversible sentences, Ss took no longer to judge the irreversible passive
The flowers are being watered by the girl than the equivalent irreversible active *The girl is watering the flowers*, despite the fact that the
passive is supposed to need an extra transformation. With reversible
sentences subjects did take longer to judge passives than actives.

SAQ 9
Which of these sentences (taken from Herriot, 1969) should subjects find easy or difficult?
(a) *The doctor treated the patient.*
(b) *The boy was kissed by the girl.*
(c) *The lifeguard was saved by the bather.*

Since 1965, Chomsky has continued to dominate linguistics in the sense that even linguists who think of themselves as anti-Chomsky have implicitly accepted his views about the aims of linguistic theory. Chomsky's later reformulations of linguistic competence are of great interest to linguists but have had little impact on psychological theories of language. This is mainly due to a belated recognition of crucial differences between a linguistic competence theory and psychological models of performance.

Summary of Section 3

- Chomsky's transformational grammar specifies syntactic rules which reflect linguistic competence, as demonstrated by speakers' ability to distinguish between grammatical and ungrammatical sentences.
- There are two types of rules: rewriting rules, which generate syntactic tree structures for sentences, and transformational rules, which produce passives and negatives.
- In Chomsky's 1965 theory, the syntax component generates deep structures and surface structures. Deep structures contain the syntactic information necessary for interpretation by the semantics component. Surface structures contain the syntactic information necessary for the phonological component to represent the sounds of words in the correct order. The three components in Chomsky's theory are independent, allowing for no interaction between syntactic and semantic analysis.
- Psycholinguists interpreted Chomsky's 1965 theory as a model for the production of sentences but experiments showed that people do not complete a full syntactic analysis of sentences before starting to interpret meanings (see Techniques Box A).

4   *Semantic representations*

Semantics describes the way in which the meanings of sentences are represented. **Sentence representations** are built up from combinations of the meanings of words. This may seem a relatively easy task until one remembers that many words have more than one meaning. Semantic representations have to take into account the potential representations of lexical items, combining them according to the rules of syntax. In Section 2, three different representations of lexical items were presented.

SAQ 10
Write down the names of the three ways of representing word meanings in the lexicon.

The aim of each of these three theories about lexical representations is to provide a basis for selecting appropriate word meanings in order to build up meaningful representations of sentences. The general idea is to specify which combinations of words make sense. These rules are known as **selection restrictions** because they select semantically acceptable sentence representations. Let's now consider each of the main types of lexical representations to evaluate their success in generating semantic representations of sentences by putting into operation selection restrictions that rule out unacceptable semantic representations.

4.1   Semantic features and semantic representations

Start by looking back at Section 2.2 which describes semantic feature lexical representations. Selection restrictions can be formulated by referring to semantic features which rule out many different nonsensical combinations. A single rule which states that all adjectives which have the feature (+ state of mind) are not allowed to be combined with objects with the feature (– human) rules out many combinations like *despairing table, happy needle, conscientious banana.*

SAQ 11
(a) What semantic features might be needed to define possible subjects of the verb *admire*?
(b) What semantic features might be needed to define possible objects of *admire*?

To see how selection restrictions work, let us take as an example a sentence like *He hit the ball.* The word 'hit' would have a list of features indicating that it has two possible senses:
1 The sense of 'strike' with an instrument, which requires (+ human) as subject and (+ physical object) for both instrument and object (e.g. *The man hit the ball with a bat*).
2 The sense of 'collide' which can refer to any two physical objects (e.g. *The rock hit the car*).

SAQ 12
Looking at the definitions given above for *hit*, indicate which of the following sentences are acceptable and why:
(a) *Peter hit the rock with a ball.*
(b) *The car hit a truck with a ball.*
(c) *A rock hit Peter.*
(d) *John hit Peter at the ball.*

The acceptability of sentence (d) raises some problems for semantic feature theories. It is not easy to see how the fact that a dance is a place where things like hitting can occur can be incorporated into the semantic features of the individual word 'dance'. The 'dance' sense of 'ball' in Figure 1.1 (see Section 2.2) would need to have features specifying all possible occurrences which could take place at a dance. Another problem with attaching semantic features to individual words is that the same features would have to be repeated for all words with a similar meaning; 'dance', 'ball', 'party', 'rave-up', 'race meeting', 'wedding' would all have to be defined as social activities where things can happen. This would result in very complex feature lists for each word in the lexicon, each of which would have to be combined to produce acceptable semantic representations of sentences.

4.2   Case frames and semantic representations

Start by looking back at Section 2.3, which describes lexical representations in terms of semantic cases.

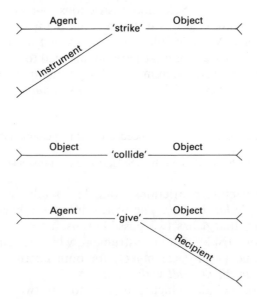

Figure 1.7   Case frames for verbs

The diagrams in Figure 1.7 represent **case frames** for verbs. Each case frame specifies **case slots** which have to be filled in by appropriate cases. Thus, the 'strike' sense of *hit* would be defined as needing an Agent, an Object and a possible optional Instrument. The 'collide' sense of *hit* would be defined as requiring two Objects because both the objects involved in a collision are affected by the action expressed by the verb. The selection of words to fill these case slots should result in an appropriate semantic representation of a sentence. Selection restrictions operate by defining the sentence case frames in which verbs can appear. The main disadvantage of a case-frame analysis is that it does not give any information about the types of words which can fulfill the case slots. There is nothing to prevent an unsuitable Object and Instrument being selected for the 'strike' sense of *hit*, as in *John hit the Rocky Mountains with a pencil*.

4.3   Semantic primitives and semantic representations

Start by looking back to Section 2.4 which describes semantic primitives as lexical representations. In order to represent the meanings of sentences, Schank's Acts are expressed in terms of case frames just like the semantic cases. The essential difference is that, instead of specifying case frames for all the individual words in the lexicon, Schank only needs to provide one case frame for each primitive action.

As an example, the 'strike' and 'collide' meanings of *hit* would be represented by the following case frames for primitive actions:

'strike'
Actor: human (possibly using instrument)
Act: PROPEL
Object: physical object

'collide'
Actor: none
Act: PTRANS
Objects: at least two physical objects

The case slots for each Act would have to be filled in with appropriate words to arrive at an acceptable semantic representation of a sentence. All verbs like *strike, hit, kick, throw* would be analysed as case frames for PROPEL. All verbs which mean collide can be analysed as appropriate case frames for PTRANS, the primitive Act which is defined as the physical transfer of an object from one location to another, in this case towards another object.

You will find it instructive to compare this primitive Act case frame format with the other representations for 'strike' and 'collide' — as semantic feature selection restrictions in Section 4.1 and as semantic case frames for verbs in Section 4.2. All these formats represent the same information about possible subjects and objects, but the semantic primitives approach has the additional advantage that the case frame for 'strike' also applies to all other verbs which involve applying force to a physical object (PROPEL).

Despite these advantages, Schank's theory comes up against the same problems as other semantic theories based on lexical meanings. In particular, there is the difficulty of specifying the fine grain of which word combinations make sense. For instance, it would be necessary to list all the objects which are 'giveable' in order to exclude very odd sentences like *John gave Mary the Rocky Mountains*.

A second drawback is that to reduce words (e.g. *say, joke, preach, threaten, read*) to a single MTRANS primitive act obviously loses a lot of information.

On the positive side, the use of primitives does make it possible to express similarities between all words which involve ATRANS, like *give, take, sell, buy*, or all words which involve INGEST, like *eat, breathe, drink*. This leads to an economy of selection restrictions because the constraints for all words for transferring mental information can be expressed just once for the primitive MTRANS (i.e. that they all require human Actors and Recipients).

4.4 Syntax or semantics?

So far, we have discussed semantic representations of sentences without considering the role of syntax. Whichever type of lexical representation is being considered, it is still necessary to take into account syntactic rules for combining individual words. An active sentence, *John hit the ball*, and the equivalent passive sentence, *The ball was hit by John*, would both be mapped on to the same semantic representation. But it is knowledge of the syntactic rules for transforming active sentences into passives which allows the 'deep structure' of both sentences to be given the same semantic analysis. The issue which has exercised psychologists is whether syntactic parsing to produce a syntactic tree structure showing grammatical relations between words is necessary for deciding on the semantic representations of a sentence.

Supporters of the need for syntactic structures assume that a syntactic structure will be generated in terms of syntactic symbols like NP, VP, etc. Those who take the semantic position deny the need for syntactic rules. Instead, they believe that semantic information about word meanings in the lexicon is sufficient to derive semantic representations of sentences.

Ritchie and Thompson (1984) give amusing caricatures of how the semantic approach and the syntactic approach would interpret a potentially ambiguous sentence like *Robin banks with Barclays*:

> A caricature of the semantic position proceeds as follows:
> My dictionary (i.e. lexicon) tells me that this string of characters either refers to the edges of bodies of water, to financial institutions, or to the process of using a financial institution. Similarly, it tells me that *Robin* refers to a human, and *Barclays* to a particular financial institution. There is only one sensible way of combining these meanings into a single coherent meaning — The human named Robin uses the financial institution named Barclays.
> A caricature of the syntactic position would be:
> My dictionary (of syntactic rules) tells me that *Robin* is a proper noun, *banks* either a plural noun or the third person singular of a verb, *with* a preposition and *Barclays* another proper noun. My grammar tells me that well-formed utterances in English can consist of the sequence proper noun, verb, preposition, proper noun but that the sequence proper noun, noun, preposition, proper noun is not a well-formed English utterance. Therefore *banks* is in this case a verb.

As Ritchie and Thompson go on to point out, both approaches have advantages and disadvantages. The first takes us nearer to the actual meaning of the sentence but the second specifies precise syntactic rules. Semantic analysis depends on knowing that there is 'only one sensible way of combining word meanings into a single coherent meaning'. But this is not necessarily always the case. Some sentences have more than one sensible meaning (e.g. *The bank has collapsed*). It is clear that we don't yet know enough about how we extract semantic representations which reflect both syntactic and semantic knowledge.

Summary of Section 4

- Semantic representations of sentences are derived from a combination of lexical representations of the meanings of the words in the sentence. Selection restrictions operate to distinguish between unacceptable and meaningful combinations of words.
- Selection restrictions can be represented in terms of permissible combinations of semantic features.
- Case frames specify the types of words which are acceptable to fill case slots.
- Primitive acts can be specified in terms of case frames for all verbs which are examples of a limited number of Acts.
- The extent to which syntactic information and semantic information are both necessary for understanding sentences is still controversial.

5 *Representations of discourse*

So far we have been considering representations of individual words and individual sentences. But, of course, most of what we read consists of longer passages of text, newspaper articles, letters, short stories, novels and biographies. These are collectively termed **discourse**. This section will explore the issue of how the semantic representations of individual sentences are combined to arrive at a coherent representation when they are embedded in a larger discourse.

5.1 *Story grammars*

One suggestion is that people have stored in memory representations of the typical structures of texts, especially when reading stories. The basic notion is that we know something about how stories are structured, over and above the content of any particular story. The only way we can know this is from experiences of hearing and reading many stories, all of which conform to a typical structure.

When you think of all the different kinds of stories you may have read — novels, collections of short stories, children's stories, newspaper stories — you may well wonder if there are any rules which can define a single typical structure for all stories. Several psychologists have proposed that, at least for traditional stories, all the different 'surface' forms of stories can be interpreted in terms of a 'deep' underlying structure which is universal to all stories. This deep structure can be defined by a set of rules known as a **story grammar**. Let us take a simple story as an example (each phrase in the story is identified by a number):

Once upon a time (1) *a prince and princess* (2) *were walking in the forest* (3). *The prince wanted to marry the princess* (4). *He asked her to marry him* (5). *She said yes* (6). *They got married and lived happily ever after* (7).

Figure 1.8 shows how story grammar rules can be used to generate a tree structure for this particular story. Each element is rewritten as other elements. For example, a story is rewritten at the next level as a Setting, Theme, Plot and Resolution. The Setting can be further rewritten as Characters, Location and Time, which are then rewritten as the actual words of the story. Note that the idea of rewrite rules for generating tree structures in a story grammar is in exactly the same format as Chomsky's rewrite rules for generating trees for representing the syntactic structures of sentences. In fact, this is the reason why this way of representing stories is known as a story grammar.

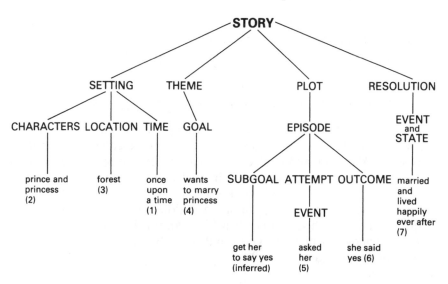

Figure 1.8   Tree structure for a simple story

Mandler and Johnson (1977) made the point that story grammars are particularly suitable for folk-tales which are passed on orally from generation to generation before being written down. The reason why traditional story-tellers are able to recite long complex stories from memory is that the stories conform to an underlying structure in which a single protagonist carries out a series of actions to achieve a stated goal. Regardless of how many events occur in the story, a teller can keep track of the overall framework of the story. It has often been noted that story-tellers produce slightly different versions of a basic story on each occasion, showing that they have memorized, not a word-perfect surface version, but rather the underlying deep structure which enables them to generate the events in the story.

Naturally, there are many other kinds of stories besides traditional folk-tales. Particularly when stories are written for reading at leisure, elements may deliberately be omitted or distorted in order to surprise, as in mystery stories. Nevertheless, as readers we often feel cheated if a story does not resolve itself into some kind of satisfactory conclusion. We also have memory schemas which represent our expectations about other types of text with very different conventions: for instance, history books, reports of scientific experiments, or airline timetables.

Black and Wilensky (1979) have argued that there is no need to postulate special story grammars. All that is necessary is an under-standing of people's goals and motivations in real-life situations. Since stories are about people, they will naturally describe people's usual behaviour. If you look back to the story grammar tree in Figure 1.8, you will see that the prince and princess story could also be analysed as representing motivations and actions:

GOAL   Prince wants to marry princess

ACTION   Asks princess to marry him

SUCCESS   They marry and live happily ever after

It is certainly not at all easy to disentangle story schemas from our general knowledge about goals and actions. Some cognitive psychologists (e.g. Van Dijk and Kintsch, 1983) accept the compromise position that both are involved. There are indeed literary conventions governing stories and other kinds of texts irrespective of content. We do expect stories to have a beginning, a middle and an end and to deal with characters and situations. But how can this be distinguished from our knowledge of people's goals and plans based on our own experiences of the world about us?

5.2   Representations of events as scripts

Many stories and conversations refer to events which are well understood. Schank and his colleagues (Schank and Abelson, 1977) have developed a theory that typical events can be represented as **scripts**. One well-known example is the Restaurant Script shown in Figure 1.9. The basic idea is that storing a script in memory enables a language user to make sense of stories which relate to typical events.

TECHNIQUES BOX B

Bower, Black and Turner's Experiments (1979)

Rationale
The idea behind these experiments was to test whether people would agree about which events occur in particular scripts.

Method
Bower et al. asked subjects to write lists of actions people would normally perform in certain situations, like going to a restaurant, attending a lecture and visiting a doctor.

Results
When the lists of actions produced by subjects for each script situation were compared, a great deal of agreement was found about the main events. For instance, attending a lecture involves entering a room, finding a seat, taking out a notebook, taking notes, checking the time, and — possibly with a feeling of relief — leaving at the end.

Name: Restaurant

Props: Tables	*Roles:* Customer
Menu	Waiter/waitress
Food	Cook
Bill	Cashier
Money	Owner
Tip	

Entry conditions: Customer is hungry	*Results:* Customer has less money
Customer has money	Owner has more money
	Customer is not hungry

Scene 1: Entering
    Customer enters restaurant
    Customer looks for table
    Customer decides where to sit
    Customer goes to table
    Customer sits down

Scene 2: Ordering
    Waitress brings menu
    Customer reads menu
    Customer decides on food
    Customer orders food
    Waitress gives food order to cook
    Cook prepares food

Scene 3: Eating
    Cook gives food to waitress
    Waitress brings food to customer
    Customer eats food

Scene 4: Exiting
    Customer asks for bill
    Waitress gives bill to customer
    Customer gives tip to waitress
    Customer goes to cashier
    Customer gives money to cashier
    Customer leaves restaurant

Figure 1.9   Restaurant script (adapted from Bower, Black and Turner, 1979)

Some experiments which tested whether people represent routine events as mental scripts which incorporate the actions which are likely to occur are described in Techniques Box B opposite.

SAQ 13
Write down some actions which you think should be included in a 'Getting up in the morning' script.

In another experiment, Bower et al. read out to subjects short stories about script-based events. An example would be:

> *The patient visited his doctor and waited in the waiting room. He went in to see the doctor who gave him some pills.*

After a brief interval, subjects were asked to write down what they had heard. The results showed that the subjects remembered the sentences in the story but they also wrote down some other actions (e.g. that the patient had spoken to the receptionist or read a magazine while waiting) which had not been stated in that particular story. One conclusion that can be drawn from these results is that subjects were making inferences about events which are likely to occur in a 'doctor' script even though these actions were not explicitly mentioned in the story.

Bower and his colleagues also drew attention to the fact that, after experiencing several events of a similar type, people combine individual scripts into more general superordinate scripts which contain the events common to all visits to professionals. It is these more general scripts which lead to expectations about actions which are equally likely to occur in the waiting rooms of doctors, dentists, chiropodists and lawyers. This proposal appears to cut down the need for an enormous proliferation of individual scripts for each type of event. Actions which are common to many events can be incorporated into general scripts (e.g. visiting all types of offices, waiting to be seen, paying for all services). It is argued that this kind of general script-based knowledge is necessary for understanding language at the discourse level.

5.3   *Representations of texts as macrostructures*

When reading a long text, most people cannot remember the actual wording in each sentence. Instead, they recall only the main gist of the text, leaving out less important details. Van Dijk and Kintsch (1983) use the term **macrostructure** to represent the gist of the text which is remembered.

One method for studying macrostructures is to ask subjects to make summaries of texts. Van Dijk and Kintsch (1983) quote studies which found that, at their first attempts at summarizing a text, subjects included many elaborative details. It was only in later attempts that details were eliminated so as to produce a short summary emphasizing the main points.

One important point that needs to be stressed is that each reader may end up with a different macrostructure for the same text, depending on his or her attitudes and beliefs about the topic being discussed. Two people who disagree about politics may go away with quite different macrostructures of a political speech. Years after reading a novel like *War and Peace*, the macrostructure stored in your memory may only contain the information that there are a lot of battles and a family with a charming girl called Natasha. Certainly, I have a composite macrostructure for the plots of Agatha Christie stories; it is only when I start reading one of them that specific details about setting and plot remind me that I may have read this one before.

The emphasis on the prior knowledge of each particular reader brings us round full circle to the issue of general knowledge versus linguistic knowledge. The analysis of larger units of language, like stories and scripts, depends on general knowledge and expectations about the world. Furthermore, the macrostructures we store in memory themselves add to the knowledge we can bring to bear on the next text we read. The accumulated knowledge we gain from language results from our interpretations of everything we hear and read.

5.4   The effort after meaning: making inferences

It is obvious from the discussion in the previous section that language users do not attempt to interpret a discourse with a clean slate. They are continually making inferences in an effort to make sense of what they hear and read, based on their general knowledge and expectations.

Clark (1977) claimed that listeners can only understand texts if they have prior knowledge of the topic under discussion. When there is no direct reference to the topic, people fill the gap by making **bridging inferences**. These are called bridging inferences because they construct a 'bridge' between something that is already known and some new information. A classic example given by Clark is *John put the picnic things in the car. The beer was warm.*

SAQ 14
(a) What bridging inference about the contents of the picnic must be made to understand the second sentence?
(b) What general knowledge is likely to be involved in finding this an acceptable statement?

Sometimes, of course, bridging inferences intended by the speaker are not the same as those assumed by the listener. Take the sentence: *John was dancing with Susan when Mary left the party early.* This would be easy to understand if both speaker and hearer knew the past history of the three characters in order to make bridging inferences based on prior knowledge. The inference that Mary might be annoyed by John choosing to dance with Susan is based on a knowledge-based stereotype of male/female relationships. It is equally plausible, however, that John and Susan are married and that Mary left because she was ill. Understanding depends on shared assumptions about social conventions. Misunderstandings arise when mutual general knowledge and beliefs break down.

A classic experiment by Bransford and Johnson (1972) demonstrates how necessary it is to have prior knowledge of what topic is being discussed in order to understand a text (see Techniques Box C).

TECHNIQUES BOX C
Bransford and Johnson's Experiment (1972)

Rationale

The authors argue that people are more likely to be able to comprehend and remember a passage of text if they know what it is about. If the appropriate knowledge is not available, people will not be able to make sense of what they hear and will therefore remember very little of it.

Method

Subjects listened to the following passage:

> The procedure is actually quite simple. First you arrange things into different groups. Of course one pile may be sufficient depending on how much there is to do. If you have to go somewhere else due to lack of facilities that is the next step, otherwise you are pretty well set. It is important not to overdo things. That is, it is better to do too few things at once than too many. In the short run this may not seem important but complications can easily arise. A mistake can be expensive as well. At first the whole picture will seem complicated. Soon, however, it will become just another fact of life. It is difficult to foresee any end to the necessity for this task in the immediate future, but then one never can tell. After the procedure is completed one arranges the materials into different groups again. Then they can be put into their appropriate places. Eventually they will be used once more and the whole cycle will then have to be repeated. However, that is a part of life.

Try this for yourself. Put your hand over the passage and see how much you can remember about it. Now read the passage again but with the additional information that the topic is 'Washing Clothes'.

In Bransford and Johnson's experiment the passage was read out to subjects either with no title, or the title 'Washing Clothes' was presented before hearing the text, or the title was presented after hearing the text but before recall. Subjects were asked to recall the text and also to rate it for comprehensibility.

Results

Mean comprehension ratings and recall scores:

	No title	Title before	Title after
Comprehension ratings	2.29	4.50	2.12
Recall scores	2.82	5.83	2.65

Comprehension and recall scores were much better for the group who had been given the title before hearing the passage. Note that giving subjects the title after they had already heard the passage did not help them to recall the text.

The knowledge that the topic of the passage is washing clothes enables the listener to make inferences which 'make sense' of the bits about 'going somewhere else if there is a lack of facilities' and the 'arrangement of materials into different piles', and so on. Of course, you will realize that the experimenters chose the passage very cleverly so as to give no clues which would give away what it was about. Did you nevertheless try to impose some interpretation when you first read the text?

Subjects who were not given a title would still have been attempting to understand it. In the absence of clues to indicate the topic or script, people tend to make **elaborative inferences** which they hope will turn out to be confirmed later. Examples might be to think about all possible types of objects which can be piled up. One thing seems certain: language users will go to any lengths in their effort after meanings. It is simply not possible to read or listen to discourse without trying to make inferences which will bridge the gap between understanding or not understanding.

Summary of Section 5

- Story grammars define rules for representing the structures of typical stories.
- Knowledge of goals and plans for action underlie the understanding of stories about human actions.
- Schank and his colleagues proposed that typical events can be represented as scripts (e.g. the Restaurant Script), and that these can be helpful in understanding descriptions of probable events.
- Readers derive macrostructures for longer texts by eliminating unnecessary details.
- Prior knowledge aids language understanding through bridging inferences and elaborative inferences in order to achieve meaningful interpretations of a discourse.

6   Some conclusions

The main topic of Part I has been to outline representations of knowledge relevant to understanding language. Section 2 considered three ways of representing word meanings in the lexicon: semantic features, semantic cases and semantic primitives. In Section 3, representations of syntactic rules were described, reflecting the influence of Chomsky's theory of syntactic competence. Section 4 tackled the difficult topic of how semantic representations of sentences are arrived at on the basis of the selection restrictions built into lexical meanings. A question was raised about the need for deriving syntactic structures when understanding sentences.

Finally, in Section 5, the many factors which influence representations of whole texts and other types of discourse were discussed. Story grammars and scripts emphasize the importance of general knowledge in making bridging inferences about the situations and topics in discourse.

At the level of discourse representations, it is particularly difficult to separate out knowledge of a language from general knowledge of the world. Schank, and many others, believe that representations of real-life knowledge (scripts) are used to interpret all inputs, whether they are actual experiences, words or texts. People are continually exploiting their knowledge of situations and events to make inferences and construct interpretations of the world around them. There is no essential difference between making sense of an actual visit to the doctor and reading a story about visiting a doctor. Humans activate their general knowledge about situations and events in order to make sense of linguistic descriptions. According to this view, understanding language is not a separate activity but is part of our experience of the world.

In contrast, other psychologists emphasize that linguistic knowledge is a very specialized skill. Learning the vocabulary of a language, the grammar and the rules for deriving meaningful representations of individual utterances and longer texts, is not an easy task for an adult learning a new language. Shared general knowledge of likely situations and events is undoubtedly important. But two people who do not have the same linguistic knowledge of a specific language will find it hard to communicate meaningfully. I expect you have all experienced occasions when, in the absence of a common language, all communication is reduced to an attempt to express your intended meaning by gestures which may easily be misunderstood. This is evidence in favour of the need for a specialized linguistic competence which represents the rules and skills required to speak and understand a language.

A further issue is whether, even within the confines of specific linguistic competence, there are independent modules which represent lexical knowledge, syntactic knowledge and semantic knowledge. This implies that it is possible to isolate specific types of knowledge. According to this modular concept of individual linguistic representations, lexical, syntactic and semantic processing of sentences would be represented as independent modules. It would only be at the level of discourse understanding that inferences based on general knowledge about situations and events would come into play.

The opposing position is that it is impossible to isolate specific linguistic modules. The argument is that language users are able to access all types of information as they require it. Even lexical meanings may derive from knowledge of the world. We act towards tables and chairs as inanimate objects and would be astonished if they started talking to us. How can this knowledge be distinguished from our understanding of the words which represent tables and chairs? We can form an appropriate linguistic semantic representation for the sentence *Jane sat on the table*. But when faced with a sentence like *The table talked to Jane*, do we rule it out on the basis of the lexical representation of the verb *talked* or because we know that talking tables are not encountered in the real world? Many psychologists support the view that all types of knowledge stored in memory are available simultaneously. In Part II the contrast between independent linguistic modules as opposed to a more interactive approach will be a major theme.

Further reading

Psycholinguistics: Central Topics by Alan Garnham (1985) provides a very thorough account of all the main topics covered in Part I.

Schank has written an interesting little book, *Reading and Understanding* (1982), in which he presents his theories about scripts in the form of guidance to teachers of reading.

For more information about Noam Chomksy's theory and its impact on psychology you can consult *Psycholinguistics: Chomksy and Psychology* by Greene (1972) or *Thinking and Language* by Greene (1975).

There is an interesting discussion of the issues involved in the relationship between language and thought in *The Psychology of Cognition* by Cohen (1983), which includes evidence about the ability of animals to learn language and compares the cognitive development of hearing and deaf children.

Part II
Language Processes and Models

Judith Greene

Part II Language Processes and Models

Contents

1   Introduction   53
1.1 Modular models   54
1.2 A linear model   54
1.3 An interactive model   55
1.4 Methods of investigation   57

2   Lexical processing and semantic processing   58
2.1 Semantic priming experiments   59
2.2 Cross-modal semantic priming experiments   60
2.3 The role of the lexicon in computer models   65
2.4 Cottrell's lexically-based model   67

3   Syntactic processing and semantic processing   69
3.1 Grammatical judgements   70
3.2 Effects of syntactic priming   70
3.3 The role of syntactic parsers in computer models   73
3.4 Winograd's interactive model of language understanding   78

4   Discourse processing and general knowledge   81
4.1 General knowledge inferences: scripts revisited   82
4.2 St John's story gestalt model   83

5   Concluding issues   87

Further reading   89

1   *Introduction*

The types of linguistic knowledge described in Part I can be thought of as 'sources of information' available to anyone who knows a language. These were described as representations of knowledge stored in the brain: knowledge of the lexicon, syntax, semantics and discourse. Part II will consider the same knowledge representations as were described in Part I. However, Part II will ask questions about how the different types of linguistic knowledge are actually used to recognize words and understand grammatically correct meaningful sentences in discourse (i.e. in texts, stories and conversations). In other words, what kinds of *processes* are involved in language understanding?

The representations discussed in Part I were treated as types of information stored in memory. In Part II the emphasis will be on how linguistic outputs are processed in order to build up linguistic representations of sentences and texts. The cognitive system which carries out linguistic processing in the brain is thought of as a **language processor**. This language processor has access to appropriate memory stores of knowledge, including the lexicon, syntax and semantics.

At the end of Part I, reference was made to two opposing views of how the language processor works. The alternatives are that the language processor consists of separate independent linguistic modules or, on the other hand, that it operates in an interactive mode in which linguistic and general knowledge are available at all stages of the language understanding process.

Another way of expressing this distinction is to ask whether there are several *levels* of understanding corresponding to the different stages of processing or whether language understanding is a unitary process. Are the *outputs* of the language processor in the form of semantic representations of individual sentences or are they macrostructure representations of whole texts? This is a point you should bear in mind when considering the evidence for different models of the language processor. Because semantic understanding is the aim of all language processing, in Part II the different levels of language processing will be discussed in relation to their influence on the semantic processes involved in language understanding.

Another important question is whether the language understanding process is identical for both spoken and written speech. Most of the examples of discourse have been of written texts, and stories. And yet a great deal of language consists of spoken conversations. It is usually assumed that the language processor, which incorporates knowledge of the vocabulary and grammar of a language, is common to the comprehension of both spoken and written inputs. However, language understanding in its wider sense of comprehending discourse may have different characteristics depending on whether the input is written or spoken. Spoken language may convey meanings in different ways, relying on intonation and stress, signalling an understanding of a speaker's intentions and allowing for immediate feedback in a particular situation. Written texts are usually read in isolation and so have to be more self-explanatory and complete, which we hope is true of this book that you are now in the process of reading. Most of the theories of language discussed in this volume are concerned with written language. But you will notice that, in some of the experiments reported in the Techniques Boxes, subjects are required to listen to spoken inputs.

SAQ 15
What advantages of speech as a mode of communication may be lost when talking on the telephone?

1.1   Modular models

Theories of linguistic processing have traditionally been formulated within an **information processing framework**. This assumes that there is a flow of information from linguistic inputs through various processing stages resulting in a final output which represents language comprehension. The processing stages can be thought of as separate **linguistic modules**: for example, a lexical module, a syntactic module, a semantic module and a discourse module. This is why such models are known as modular models.

Within the modular framework, it is still possible to ask the question whether each module operates independently or whether it is possible for processing in one module to be influenced by processing in other modules. It is also reasonable to investigate whether processing by one module can be influenced by simultaneously accessing different kinds of knowledge stored in memory.

Thus, there are two main models for considering how humans process language. In the *linear model*, the processing modules are separate stages which are carried out one at a time. In the *interactive model*, the processing involved in several modules can occur simultaneously, allowing different types of knowledge to interact, including both linguistic knowledge and general knowledge of the world. These models will be described more fully in the next two sections.

1.2   A linear model

The essence of this type of model is that each type of processing is completed before the next stage starts. Figure 2.1 shows the modules as independent processing stages. The arrows going from left to right demonstrate that information can only travel in one direction from each processing stage to the next, starting with the initial input of words and ending with the final outputs which signal language understanding. The single arrow from each kind of knowledge in memory indicates that each type of knowledge can only affect a single processing stage.

Figure 2.1 can be described as a **linear model** because it consists of a line of processing stages, each of which has to be completed before the next stage can come into operation. This implies that each stage is independent of every other stage. It can also be thought of as involving **bottom-up processing** because the initial processing of inputs occurs without being influenced by 'higher' types of knowledge.

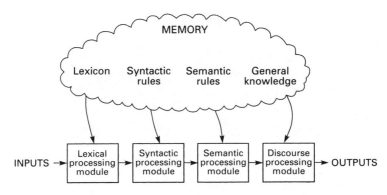

Figure 2.1 A linear model of language processing

It has been argued that linear models are 'cognitively efficient' because the brain may have evolved to allow for fast processing by independent sub-systems for such processes as recognizing words and visual recognition of faces. The argument is that these initial modules can operate faster on their own just because they do not have to take account of the products of slower high-level processing, such as, for example, the contribution of general knowledge in understanding discourse. According to this model, language understanding would be the end result of rapid automatic processing of word meanings and syntactic processing.

1.3   An interactive model

An interactive model implies that the various types of knowledge implicated in the processing modules are all available at the same time and can be brought in at any point to aid language understanding.

Figure 2.2 shows an interactive model. In this model the arrows between the processing modules provide links so that the modules can interact with each other's inputs and outputs. The downward arrows from the types of knowledge in memory indicate that each type of knowledge can influence more than one processing module. Figure 2.2 can be described as an **interactive model** because different types of knowledge from other modules can interact with each other. It can be thought of as involving **top-down processing** because 'higher' knowledge influences the bottom-up processing of linguistic inputs. Processing in an interactive model is multidirectional — rather than unidirectional as in the linear model.

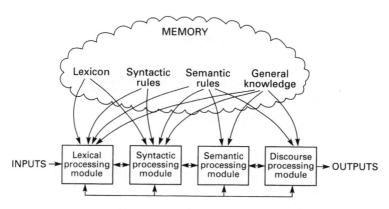

Figure 2.2 An interactive model of language processing

It has also been argued that interactive models are more 'cognitively efficient'. Because more information is available at any one time, processing can be speeded up by taking into account all the relevant information. For instance, suppose you are trying to understand the potentially ambiguous sentence, *Visiting aunts can be a nuisance.* Processing the words on their own could produce two possible meanings: either that having to visit aunts is a nuisance or that aunts who visit you are a nuisance. This ambiguity would be expected to slow down understanding. But knowing that the sentence has been uttered in the context of *Aunt Jane and Aunt Dottie dropped in unexpectedly last week* would certainly make it easier to select the appropriate sentence meaning. The argument is that a system which allows general knowledge and context to interact with and influence language processing will produce a faster and more accurate interpretation of sentences.

The rest of Part II will be structured around these two models. In each section, processing stages will be analysed in order to investigate whether they operate as independent stages or whether they can be demonstrated to interact in such a way that more than one kind of information is currently influencing linguistic processing. In other words, do people first recognize words in the lexicon, and only then analyse syntactic structures, and, only after these processes are completed, take into account sentence meanings and finally general knowledge? Or are all these sources of knowledge simultaneously invoked when processing language?

1.4   Methods of investigation

It is obvious from the discussion so far that arguments about cognitive efficiency can be employed to support both the linear model and the interactive model. So the next step must be to consider what kinds of evidence could be used to decide between the linear and interactive models. The first source of evidence comes from experiments which are designed to investigate the factors which affect the processing of linguistic inputs. Since understanding language is such a rapid and automatic process, experiments which investigate the fine details of linguistic processing have to be very ingenious in order to tap language processing as it occurs.

In each section, experiments will be described and evaluated with reference to deciding between linear and interactive models. One interesting point to watch out for is whether there are any differences between immediate processing of sentences *as they occur* (also known as **on-line processing**), and the more **delayed processing** which is based on understanding *completed* sentences and texts.

Experiments are not the only method for studying language comprehension. During the 1970s and into the 1980s a lot of faith and effort were put into developing computer programs which would be able to understand language (Greene, 1986). **Computer models** have so far failed to simulate more than a small fraction of human understanding, either providing a superficial mimicry of human responses, or getting bogged down in attempting to represent all the knowledge needed to understand just a few sentences. Other more recent computer models, which claim to be based more closely on the working of the human brain, are still limited to very small domains of knowledge.

Nevertheless, despite these apparent failures, the ideas used in developing computer models of language have provided revealing insights about their potential and their limitations for studying language understanding. There will be references to the principles underlying computer models in most sections of Part II.

Summary of Section 1

- Part I introduced different types of knowledge involved in language understanding; Part II is concerned with how such knowledge is used in processing language.
- The linear model represents language processing as separate and independent processing modules, each of which has to be completed before the next module can come into operation.
- The interactive model represents language processing as involving interaction between modules and sources of knowledge.
- Major methodologies include experiments designed to tap on-line language processes while they are occurring and computer programs designed to simulate human language processes.

2 Lexical processing and semantic processing

It is natural to think of individual words as the building blocks for understanding sentences. The contrast here is between models in which the recognition of word meanings is a separate, independent lexical processing module and models which see word meanings as depending on the sentence context in which they appear and so requiring interactive processing between the lexical and semantic modules. The question to be discussed in this section is whether the identification of possible meanings for words takes place as a separate, independent module or whether lexical meanings can only be selected in an interactive context which takes into account the semantic meanings of whole sentences.

The first issue to consider is whether it is possible to specify the meanings of individual words in isolation. As indicated in Part I, Section 4, the word *hit* has several possible related meanings: for example, to strike (a ball); to collide; *hit* in *hitman*. Other words have quite separate meanings (e.g. *bug* as an insect, *bug* as a minute microphone). To bug someone can either mean to annoy (like an insect) or to spy on them (by secretly installing a device in their telephone). Words like *saw* can be a noun or a verb as in *I saw the carpenter pick up the saw* and *The carpenter began to saw*. So how can deciding on the appropriate lexical meaning of a word be an independent processing stage?

The contrast between the independent and interactive processing of lexical meanings can be phrased in terms of whether interaction occurs between the lexical and semantic modules. In the linear model shown in Figure 2.1, the two modules are shown as independent. In Figure 2.2, there is the possibility of interaction which would allow the semantic processing module to play a role in selecting appropriate word meanings from the lexicon. The experiments in the next two sections will investigate the linear independent model versus the interactive model of lexical processing.

2.1   Semantic priming experiments

The aim of semantic priming experiments is to investigate whether word meanings are accessed by an independent processing module or whether the processing of semantic context can influence lexical access. The essential feature of the **semantic priming** technique is that it tests whether it is easier to respond to a word when that word is in a relevant semantic context than when the word is in an irrelevant or inappropriate context.

The word to be responded to is called the **target word** (also sometimes called a **probe**). The relevant semantic context is known as the **prime** because it is designed to test whether the context has 'primed' (i.e. facilitated) the response to the target word. The measure of priming is when the response to the primed target word is faster and/or more accurate than the response to the same word when it has not been primed by a relevant semantic context. A classic semantic priming experiment is described in Techniques Box D.

TECHNIQUES BOX D

Semantic Priming Experiment
(Meyer and Schvaneveldt, 1971)

Rationale
The aim is to test whether a relevant semantic priming context facilitates the response to a target word. The prediction is that the response to the target word will be primed when preceded by a relevant word context (the prime) as compared with the response to the same target word in the presence of a semantic context which is not relevant (i.e. a neutral word context).

Method
The task is to read the context word and when it disappears to respond as quickly as possible to the target word. There are two types of decision which have to be made about the target word: (a) to say the word aloud (**naming task**); or (b) to press a button to indicate whether a string of letters make up a word or not (**lexical decision task**):

NAMING (saying the target word):

Context word	Target word	Response time
NURSE (prime)	DOCTOR	(FAST)
BREAD (neutral)	DOCTOR	(SLOW)

LEXICAL DECISION (deciding whether a string of letters is a word):

Context word	Target word	Response time
NURSE (prime)	DOCTOR	(FAST)
NURSE (prime)	ROTCOD	
BREAD (neutral)	DOCTOR	(SLOW)
BREAD (neutral)	ROTCOD	

Results

The outcome of this experiment demonstrates that a relevant semantic context word primes a target word by making the response to that word faster than when it is preceded by a neutral semantic context. This is found both in the naming task and in the lexical decision task.

These results have been interpreted as indicating that there is an interaction between the lexical processing and semantic processing stages. The fact that lexical access of the word *doctor* was facilitated in the context of *nurse* but not in the context of *bread* demonstrates that the lexical processes involved in naming a word or making a lexical decision were influenced by the semantic processing of a relevant semantic context.

SAQ 16

Suppose that, in another condition in the Meyer and Schvaneveldt experiment, the target word was *butter*. Write down (a) a context word which would be a priming context, and (b) a context word which would be a neutral context.

In terms of the models in Figures 2.1 and 2.2, the Meyer and Schvaneveldt experiment in Techniques Box D provides support for the interactive model. Selection of a word's meaning in the lexicon has been shown to be affected by its semantic context, even if that context is only a single word.

2.2   Cross-modal semantic priming experiments

Semantic priming was demonstrated in Techniques Box D, which supports the interactive model. So are there any arguments in favour of the linear model of independent modules? One point that has been put forward is that priming by a single word means that the priming effect could be explained away as the result of word associations. For instance, *nurse* and *doctor* are more likely to be linked in memory than *nurse* and *bread*. These word-to-word associations could be taking place in the lexical module rather than involving any semantic processing. In order to test whether the lexical and semantic modules are really independent or interactive, it is necessary for the priming context to involve the semantic processing of sentences.

Another possible explanation of Meyer and Schvaneveldt's results is that the processing of the context word had been fully completed before the target word was presented. The fully analysed lexical meaning of *nurse* was available to prime the response to *doctor*. But what would happen if the target was presented before the semantic context was fully processed? Would interaction still occur? The proposal is that lexical processing may operate as an independent processing module while a sentence is actually being processed. As indicated in Section 1.4, this is termed *on-line* processing in contrast to the *delayed* processing necessary for completed processing of the whole sentence.

Because understanding of a sentence appears to be almost instantaneous, psychologists have had to devise ingenious experimental procedures for tapping sentence processing at various stages. How can one stop a person in the middle of processing a sentence? In traditional priming experiments, both the prime word and the target word are presented in the same *modality*. Thus, in Techniques Box D the prime and target words were both seen in the visual modality (i.e. on a screen). The result is that, because they are in the same modality, the prime has to be 'wiped' before the target word can appear. It is impossible to read two words at once or to listen to two words at once. For this reason, it is impossible to investigate what would happen if the prime and target were presented simultaneously.

However, an ingenious technique was devised to enable the contextual prime and the target word to be presented simultaneously. The answer was to present one word in the auditory modality and the other in the visual modality. It has been demonstrated that saying out loud the word *nurse* still has a priming effect resulting in a faster response to the written word *doctor*. This is known as **cross-modal priming** because one of the words is in the spoken modality and the other is in the written modality. An example would be:

Nurse (spoken)   *Doctor* (written)

To recap, in the normal semantic priming technique described in Techniques Box D, it is inevitable that the prime has to come first and the target second. The advantage of cross-modal priming is that the primes and targets can be presented *simultaneously* because one is spoken and the other is written. This cross-modal methodology allows the target word to be presented at any time while the semantic context is still present. For instance, if the semantic context is the written sentence, *In the hostel the nurse was putting on her uniform*, the target word *doctor* could be spoken at any time in the preceding sentence, before or after the word *nurse*. If the target word is spoken in the middle of the written sentence, it can be assumed that the subjects will hear it while they are still processing the sentence (on-line processing). If it is spoken after the end of the sentence, the target word will occur after sentence processing has been completed (delayed processing). Using this methodology, the timing of on-line processing can be explored in detail.

Alternatively, the sentence context could be listened to over headphones and a written target word could be presented either during the sentence or after the sentence is complete. The task for the subject might be to respond by naming the target word or by deciding whether it is a word (lexical decision task — see Techniques Box D).

Examples of cross-modal priming are given below:

(a) Spoken context: *In the hostel the nurse telephoned home*
     Written target: *Doctor*
(b) Spoken context: *In the hostel the postman telephoned home*
     Written target: *Doctor*

SAQ 17
Which response to doctor would be predicted to be faster: (a) or (b)?

In the traditional semantic priming experiments, it is assumed that the prime has helped the language processor to select the target word in the lexicon faster than would be expected. The possibility of investigating on-line processing has led psychologists to consider the precise times at which lexical items may become available to the language processor.

One hypothesis which has been proposed is that, during the on-line processing of a sentence, the semantic context has not yet selected a particular lexical meaning of a word. At this early stage of processing there is access to all possible meanings of a word uninfluenced by the semantic context. It is only when semantic processing has been completed that semantic context will come into operation to select a particular word meaning.

Cross-modal priming experiments, as described in Techniques Box E, are designed to test this hypothesis by allowing target words to be presented at different times during the semantic processing of sentences. If there is evidence that none of the target words is especially facilitated during on-line processing, this indicates that all lexical meanings are equally activated. The argument is that, because the processing of semantic context has not yet had any effect on lexical processing, this is evidence in favour of independent processing by the lexical module. Without any influence from the semantic module, the lexical module automatically accesses all possible lexical meanings. This process, known as **multiple access** to the lexicon, is therefore considered as providing evidence for the linear model of independent modules.

TECHNIQUES BOX E

Cross-Modal Semantic Priming Experiment
(Seidenberg, Tanenhaus, Leiman and Bienkowski, 1982)

Rationale
This experiment was designed to discover the precise timing of the priming effect to see whether all possible meanings of a word are accessed (multiple access) independently of the sentence context in which they occur. If all lexical meanings are available, responses should be equally fast to all target words whether they are appropriate to the sentence context or not.

Method
A sentence was spoken. A written target was presented at different time intervals, either simultaneously with the last word of the sentence (0 milliseconds) or 200 milliseconds later. The task was to name the written target word as quickly as possible. Subjects were presented with a randomized set of sentences so that they would not guess the purpose of the sentences presented.

Type of context	Spoken sentence context	Written target word
Appropriate	*You should have played the spade*	CARD
Control	*You should have played the part*	CARD
Inappropriate	*Go to the store and buy a spade*	CARD
Control	*Go to the store and buy a belt*	CARD

Results
Response times for naming the target words were measured by asking subjects to speak into a microphone which measured response times in milliseconds. The amount of priming facilitation was calculated by comparing the mean naming response times to the target words in the context of each type of sentence and its control sentence.

RESPONSE TIMES (milliseconds):

Context type	0 milliseconds interval	Priming	200 milliseconds interval	Priming
Appropriate	538	18	512	20
Control	556		532	
Inappropriate	547	15	534	5
Control	562		539	

These results demonstrate that, while on-line semantic processing is still going on (0 milliseconds), priming occurs both in the appropriate context (in comparison with its control) and in the inappropriate context, as shown by the fact that the differences in response times, both in the appropriate and inappropriate condition, are nearly equal (18 and 15 milliseconds). But after the semantic processing of the sentence is completed (200 milliseconds), the naming response is primed only by the appropriate sentence context. The difference in response time for the target word in the appropriate context is now significantly different from the difference in response time for the inappropriate context (20 milliseconds compared to 5).

Results from cross-modal priming experiments have been interpreted as evidence in favour of independent processing by the lexical module. During on-line processing, all lexical meanings are equally accessible, indicating that there is multiple access to both appropriate and inappropriate lexical meanings. At this stage, semantic processing of the sentence context has no influence on lexical access. An appropriate lexical meaning is only selected after the semantic processing of the sentence context is completed.

You, the reader, who have had the opportunity to read all the priming sentences, probably find it surprising that the lexical meaning of *spade* as a gardening tool could still be available when the target word presented simultaneously is CARD. Perhaps a more plausible explanation is that, during on-line processing, the language processor has no information about semantic context and therefore responds to *spade* as an individual word regardless of the sentence context. When *spade* is presented in conjunction with the target word CARD, *spade* is primed in both the appropriate and inappropriate contexts.

This would account for the priming effects in terms of independent lexical processing but without the need to postulate multiple-access of different meanings; rather, the processor ignores the semantic context altogether. It is only after semantic processing is completed that the inappropriate context eliminates the priming effect of the 'garden tool' sense of *spade*.

SAQ 18

(a) Think of another priming sentence context which could test the hypothesis in Techniques Box E.

(*Hint*: think of a sentence which is likely to prime the selection of the lexical meaning of *spade* as a gardening implement, so that the target word *tool* would be primed.)

(b) What would be a possible control sentence?

In relation to the linear and interactive models in Figures 2.1 and 2.2, experiments like the one described in Techniques Box E indicate that during on-line processing of a sentence the lexical processing module operates independently, accessing lexical meanings with no reference to the semantic processing of sentences. It is only when semantic processing is completed that it facilitates the selection of an appropriate lexical meaning. This supports the linear model since lexical processing operates independently from the semantic processing of the sentence context, even though they are both occurring at the same time. The advantage of cross-modal semantic priming experiments is that they provide an opportunity to chart the timescale of independent and interactive processing more precisely than before.

2.3   The role of the lexicon in computer models

The semantic priming experiments in Techniques Boxes D and E demonstrate the processes involved in accessing and selecting lexical items from the pool of word meanings available in different sentence contexts. But they say little about how the lexical selection of all the words in a sentence can be used to build up an appropriate semantic representation for a whole sentence. The issue for the language processor is, given that lexical meanings have been selected, how are these lexical meanings integrated into the semantic representations of sentences?

Computer models of language understanding often incorporate representations of word meanings for the program to draw on in order to derive meaning representations of sentences and text. In Part I, three different formulations for representing the meanings of words in the lexicon were described. These were semantic features, semantic cases and semantic primitives. As was shown with the example of the different meanings of *hit*, all these theories attempt to represent the differences between all the possible meanings of words. They do this by specifying selection restrictions which restrict which word meanings can be combined to produce meaningful sentences.

By far the most commonly used formulation for representing lexical items in computer models is some form of case-frame grammar which defines verbs in terms of the Agent and Object and other case slots which are suitable for the various meanings of each verb. The purpose is to ensure that the correct lexical meaning of a word is selected to fit in with a sentence context. At this point, re-read Sections 2.3 and 4.2 in Part I to refresh your memory about the use of sentence case frames to select appropriate words to fill case slots.

One problem with case-frame representations is that the selection restrictions which determine the selection of lexical meanings are not restrictive enough. Simply to say that Agents (including animals) eat Physical Objects could lead to many unacceptable sentences being accepted by a language computer program (e.g. *John eats stones, Cows eat meat, Bees eat Christmas trees*). Equally, the rule that Agents give Physical Objects to Recipients might lead to sentences like *John gave Mary the Rocky Mountains* being processed as acceptable.

The lexical processor in a computer program needs to have detailed information about selection restrictions which enables it to, for instance, match relevant foodstuffs to particular animals.

Examples would be:

Agent = Cows	eats	Object = grass
Agent = Bees	eats	Object = nectar
Agent = John	eats	Object = foods eatable by humans
Agent = John	mows	Object = grass

As you can imagine, this would lead to the opposite problem of there being far too many selection restrictions for every verb. It seems so natural to humans that bees do not eat stones, nor people give mountains as gifts, that selection restrictions seem to be unnecessary. However, it is just because computer programs have to specify precise rules for processing linguistic inputs that they throw up problems of this kind.

SAQ 19
Write down a similar set of 'Agents' and 'Instruments' needed to fill these case slots for various games. To start you off, one example is given and you are asked to fill in the Agent and Instrument case slots for the other games listed:

Game	Agents	Instruments
CRICKET	22 men (24 with umpires)	bats ball wicket stumps
SNOOKER		
BRIDGE		
SOCCER		

2.4   Cottrell's lexically-based model

A computer program developed by Cottrell (1989) introduced the idea of **exploded cases** in order to match case slots with appropriate word meanings in sentences. In order to produce representations of sentence meanings. Cottrell developed his program in the form of lexical networks (see the example in Figure 2.3).

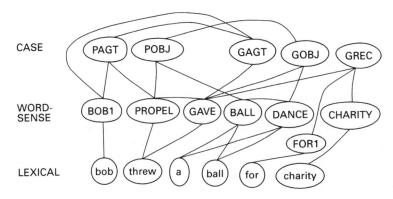

Figure 2.3   A subset of a lexical network (adapted from Cottrell, 1989)

On the top line of Figure 2.3 are the 'exploded' case frame slots labelled with selection restrictions to indicate what verbs they are suitable for. The basic idea is to represent Agents, Objects and other case slots by restricting them to words which are appropriate to the verb, as follows:

PAGT   =   Agents who can propel

POBJ   =   Objects which can be propelled

GAGT   =   Agents who can give things

GOBJ   =   Objects which can be given

GREC   =   Agents who can be recipients of gifts

The next step is to define the meanings of words (word senses) in terms of whether they are potential agents who can 'propel' or 'give' and/or possible objects of 'being propelled' or 'being given'. The middle line in Figure 2.3 gives the word senses (i.e. lexical meanings) which could fill the case slots appropriately:

BOB1   =   A particular man called Bob (Bob 2 would be used for another man called Bob)

PROPEL   =   Action of propelling

GAVE   = Action of giving

BALL   = Object which can be propelled *or* dance which can be given

CHARITY = Recipient of gifts

The final lexical stage is to test the model by getting it to match the input words to selected word meaning senses which are potential fillers for the case-frame slots. Below are examples of two sentences which might be keyed in as inputs to the computer program:

(a) *Bob threw a ball.*
(b) *Bob threw a ball for charity.*

In sentence (a), the word *Bob* is a potential filler both for PAGT (a propelling agent) and GAGT (a giving agent). The next word *threw* is likely to be selected as a PROPEL action, which results in *ball* being allocated to the POBJ case (an object which is propelled). The GIVE action is rejected. This results in a selected meaning for the sentence as *A man called Bob threw a round object.*

In sentence (b), the words *for charity* do not fit in with the PROPEL action because they do not indicate a possible location in which a physical object can be thrown. Instead, these words tip the balance for the 'give' meaning of *threw* with *a ball* filling the GOBJ case (an object which can be given) and *for charity* filling the GREC slot as the recipient of the gift. The selected meaning for this sentence is *A man called Bob gave a dance which was given to charity.* One point to notice is that in real life 'charity' is not actually an Agent who can be a 'recipient of gifts'. What is implied is that there are people running the charity who, as Agents, can receive the profits from the ball. This demonstrates the importance of making inferences in language understanding, in this case that charity balls make profits which can be handed over to human agents. These inferences are easy enough for humans but the computer program as described here would assume that 'balls' are given to 'charity'.

SAQ 20
Write down the case slots which might be filled in by the words in the sentence: *Bob threw a ball to John.* (*Hint*: You will have to add a new case for Agents who can be the recipients of propelled objects.)

When Cottrell's model is run as a computer program, all the operations run in parallel so that all the words and word senses are activated simultaneously until one selected meaning 'wins out' by filling all the case slots in the most appropriate way. Interestingly, the simultaneous activation of word inputs, word senses and lexical case frames fits in well with the notion that, during on-line processing, there is independent multiple access to a range of possible lexical meanings of words. However, the semantic processing of one selected meaning is the outcome of finding acceptable word sense fillers for a particular combination of case slots. This example demonstrates that the relationship between independent and interactive processes is a complex one.

Summary of Section 2

- Semantic priming experiments are used to investigate the effects of semantic contexts on lexical access of word meanings (see Techniques Box D).
- The results of cross-modal priming experiments show that, while a sentence context is being processed on-line, lexical processing and semantic processing operate independently (see Techniques Box E).
- Lexical meanings represented in terms of selection restrictions enable a computer program to select appropriate word meanings in order to build up semantic representations of sentences.
- Cottrell's program (1989) is designed to match appropriate word meanings to lexical case slots.

3 Syntactic processing and semantic processing

The case was made in Part 1, Section 3, for the importance of syntactic knowledge in language understanding. Without knowing the rules for ordering words and the endings which indicate the plurals of words and past and future tenses, it is impossible to understand a language fully. In the English sentence *The girl likes the boy*, word order indicates that it is the girl who likes the boy. But consider the passive sentence, *The boy is liked by the girl*. The boy is now the first noun, but the rules of English grammar still indicate that it is the girl who likes the boy. Compare *The boy with red hair is liked by the girl* and *The boy who is liked by the girl has red hair*. In the second sentence, it would be easy to assume that it is the girl who has red hair, but according to the syntactic rules of English it is still the boy who has red hair.

SAQ 21
The black dog chased by the black cat is brown.
Note down whether there is anything odd about this English sentence from the point of view of:
(a) syntax;   (b) semantics;   (c) general knowledge.

One crucial question is whether syntactic processing can be carried out in isolation from semantic processing. Is it possible to decide on a syntactic structure for a sentence without paying some attention to its meaning? In Techniques Box A in Part 1, Section 3.3, Slobin's experiment was interpreted as demonstrating that syntactic analysis can be influenced by the semantic implausibility of a sentence like *The flowers are watering the girl*. However, it has also been argued (Garnham, 1985) that this effect may only occur when the task involves a comparison between a sentence and a picture and not during on-line sentence processing. This leaves the issue of independence versus interaction between syntactic processing and semantic processing unresolved. In the rest of Section 3, the case for an independent syntactic processing module will be contrasted with evidence for interactions between syntactic and semantic processing.

3.1   Grammatical judgements

Noam Chomsky, the famous linguist whose work was described in Part I, Section 3, argued in favour of syntax as the foundation of all linguistic knowledge. He emphasized speakers' ability to judge whether sentences are grammatical regardless of their meanings. For example, *Colourless green ideas sleep furiously* can be judged as a grammatical sentence although it is a meaningless sentence. The point is that this sentence would be ruled out by a case-frame analysis indicating the kinds of agents who can sleep (i.e. most animals, but certainly not 'green ideas'). Nevertheless, the sentence conforms to the grammar of English, with the subject, verb and object in the correct order, the adjectives *colourless* and *green* modifying the noun *ideas*, while *furiously* is an adverb modifying the verb *sleep*.

The evidence from grammatical judgements supports the view that language users have the ability to separate syntactic processing from semantic processing of sentence meanings. However, these kinds of linguistic judgements are concerned with analysis of the complete sentences and so do not have any bearing on the on-line processing of sentences.

3.2   Effects of syntactic priming

Having demonstrated that people are capable of distinguishing between grammatical and non-grammatical utterances, is there other evidence that the processing of syntactic structures is an independent module? One line of investigation is to use a cross-modal priming methodology (see Techniques Box E). The results from cross-modal experiments were interpreted as demonstrating that lexical processing operates in isolation from effects of semantic processing of the sentence context.

Similar experiments have investigated whether lexical processing is independent of syntactic processing of the grammatical structure of sentence contexts. In the series of experiments reported by Seidenberg, Tanenhaus, Leiman and Bienkowksi (1982), one of the experimental conditions tested whether, during on-line processing, multiple access to possible lexical syntactic categories operates independently of the syntactic processing of sentences (see Techniques Box F). This can be thought of as a **syntactic priming experiment** because it investigates the effects of syntactic structure on the selection of lexical items which fit an appropriate syntactic category (e.g. a noun or a verb).

TECHNIQUES BOX F

Cross-modal Syntactic Priming Experiment
(Seidenberg, Tanenhaus, Leiman and Bienskowski, 1982)

Rationale
The aim is to test at different time intervals whether all possible syntactic categories are accessed simultaneously (multiple access) in sentence contexts which differ in syntactic structure. If all syntactic categories are equally available, this indicates that regardless of the effect of syntactic context, access to syntactic categories in the lexicon is independent of the syntactic structure of the sentence context. In this experiment, the sentence contexts varied in syntactic structure and the prediction was that all syntactic categories in the lexicon would be accessed during on-line processing.

Method
A sentence was spoken. A written target was presented either simultaneously with the last word of the sentence (0 milliseconds), or 200 milliseconds later. The task was to name the written target as quickly as possible. The methodology of giving subjects randomized sets of sentences was the same as in Techniques Box E.

Type of context	Spoken sentence context	Written target word
Appropriate	*They bought a rose*	FLOWER
Control	*They bought a shirt*	FLOWER
Inappropriate	*The congregation rose*	FLOWER
Control	*The congregation stood*	FLOWER

In the appropriate context, *They bought a rose*, the word *rose* is a noun and the target word *flower* is also a noun. But in the inappropriate context, *The congregation rose*, *rose* is a verb and so the noun *flower* is not an appropriate lexical selection.

Results

As in the Techniques Box E experiment, naming response times were measured in milliseconds. Priming facilitation was calculated by comparing the mean naming response times to the target words in the context of each type of sentence and its control sentence.

RESPONSE TIMES (milliseconds):

Context type	0 milliseconds interval	Priming	200 milliseconds interval	Priming
Appropriate	536	17	516	11
Control	553		527	
Inappropriate	541	12	534	-3
Control	553		531	

The results demonstrate that, while on-line syntactic processing is still going on (0 milliseconds), priming occurs both in the appropriate context and in the inappropriate context (17 and 12 milliseconds). It is only after the syntactic processing of the sentence is completed (200 milliseconds) that the naming response is primed only by the appropriate sentence context (11 compared with -3). It appears that during on-line processing the response to the target FLOWER is facilitated by the word *rose* in both the appropriate and inappropriate contexts, again demonstrating that syntactic context is ignored by the language processor.

SAQ 22

In another example, the target word *clock* was to be primed as a noun. Suppose *watch* was a good word to prime *clock* as a noun.

(a) Think of a sentence using the word *watch* which would prime *clock* as a noun.

(b) Think of a sentence also using the word *watch* which would act as a prime for a verb, and so would not prime the target *clock*.

In relation to the linear and interactive models in Figures 2.1 and 2.2, the experiment in Techniques Box F indicates that during on-line processing of a sentence the lexical processing module operates independently, accessing syntactic categories in the lexicon with no reference to the syntactic processing of sentences. It is only when the delayed syntactic processing necessary for understanding a whole sentence is completed that it facilitates the selection of an appropriate lexical syntactic category. This supports the linear model because it demonstrates that lexical and semantic processes operate independently even though they are occurring at the same time.

3.3   The role of syntactic parsers in computer models

Cross-modal priming experiments point to the independence of on-line lexical, syntactic and semantic processing. Nevertheless, it is clear that all these linguistic processes are involved in language understanding. The aim of computer models of language is to reveal all the processes involved in linguistic understanding. Many computer models include a syntactic component for analysing the syntactic structure of sentences. The linguistic processor for analysing the syntactic structures of sentences is usually called a **syntactic parser**. This reflects the, perhaps now old-fashioned, English grammar lessons which required children to 'parse' sentences into grammatical clauses and parts of speech. The argument for including a parser in a computer language program is the need to account for examples when the meaning of a sentence depends on the syntactic structure of the sentence.

Some examples are:

(i)   *The cat chased the dog.*
(ii) *Bob threw the ball to John.*
(iii) *The ball was thrown to John by Bob.*

In (i), how would the computer program know whether the cat or the dog is the Agent of *chased*? In (ii), there are two possible Agents, Bob and John, so how would the program know which to select as the Agent and which as the Recipient of the ball being thrown? Sentence (iii) is even more difficult because the Agent is at the very end of the sentence. In order to interpret these sentences, the computer program would need to know enough of the syntax of English in order to recognize the importance of word order and the syntactic significance of words like *to* and *by* to indicate that the ball is being thrown by Bob to John.

SAQ 23
(a) In the sentence *The dog, which is chasing the cat, is being chased by the bull,* would the syntactic parser decide that it is the cat or the dog which is being chased by the bull?
(b) Are there any syntactic clues to help decide which animals are chasing which other animals?

Syntactic parsers incorporate syntactic rules. The parser searches for patterns of words which indicate that they are part of a noun phrase or a verb phrase. Perhaps the most commonly used type of syntactic parser is based on a formalism known as **transition networks**, first developed by Woods (1970). They are called 'transition networks' because they look at transitions between each of the constituents of a sentence, starting at the beginning and working through the sentence from left to right. They try to construct the syntactic structure of a sentence by identifying constituents of a sentence.

The first rule of a sentence is that a sentence (S) is made up of a noun phrase (NP) and a verb phrase (VP). In Figure 2.4(a) the parser can only proceed from (S1) to (S2) if it can find an NP. From (S2) it can only finish the sentence by moving to (S3) if the next constituent it finds is a VP.

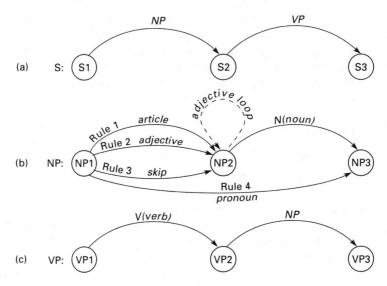

Figure 2.4   Transition networks

But how can the parser go about finding an NP? Figure 2.4(b) depicts a transition network which encapsulates most of the ways an NP can be written. The aim is to complete an NP by moving from NP1, by selecting an appropriate rule to make the transition to NP2, and finally by selecting a noun to complete the transition to end point NP3. From NP1, Rule 1 states that an article and a noun is a possible NP (e.g. *The boy*). Rule 2 states that an adjective or many adjectives (the adjective loop) are possible with or without an article (e.g. *The big boy, Many big tall boys*). Rule 3 ('skip') states that an NP can consist of a noun on its own (e.g. *John*). Finally, Rule 4 states that an NP can just be a pronoun (e.g. *He*).

SAQ 24
Which of the NP rules would generate the following NPs?
(a) *The boy*
(b) *Big blue blocks*
(c) *She*
(d) *The tall bright child*

To complete the syntactic rules for processing an NP + VP sentence, we need a transition network which searches for a verb and another NP as shown in Figure 2.4(c). Taken together, the transition networks (a), (b) and (c) in Figure 2.4 specify the rules for parsing a whole sentence. The parser works by going through the transition networks. At each transition it tries to find a word which will allow it to make a transition to the next constituent of the sentence. When the network has found a syntactic structure, by completing all the required transitions in the network, the parser reports back its successful search for the syntactic categories which make up a sentence with an acceptable syntactic structure.

Incidentally, you may have noticed that this account of how a syntactic parser works seems to incorporate many of the same syntactic rules used by Chomsky (see Part I, Section 3). The crucial difference is that Chomsky's theory was designed to describe the ideal syntactic competence required for knowledge of a language. In contrast, syntactic parsers implement the processes involved in actual language use, including strategies for dealing with incomplete and ambiguous sentences.

One question which exercises computer programmers is what action a syntactic parser should take when it is faced with the possibility of several different ways of analysing a sentence. Often it is not clear until later what the correct parse should be. For instance, if the parser came across *The old man* it would identify this as an NP. But suppose the sentence continues with the words *the boats*. The parser would have to change its analysis to *The old* (NP) *man* (V) *the boats* (NP).

There are several ways in which a parser could operate:

1 The parser could compute all possibilities at each word transition. This means that *The old* and *The old man* would both be carried forward as possible NPs. But, when you consider all the possible ways in which a sentence may end, this seems an uneconomic solution for computer or human.

2 The parser could plump for the most probable grammatical structure for an NP (e.g. *The old man*). But, if it later comes across words like *the boats*, it could back up to an earlier transition identifying *The old* as a complete NP followed by the verb *man*.

3 The parser could *look ahead* to see what is coming next before deciding how to analyse the current transition. If it sees the words *the boats* coming up it can safely identify *The old* as an NP and *man* as a verb.

4 The parser could call on a semantics component to decide the most likely interpretation of the sentence. In this case, the sentence would be equally semantically correct under either interpretation. However, if the sentence had been *The old man the tables*, the selection restrictions on combinations of word meanings would rule out the

possibility of *tables* as a possible lexical meaning for the Object case of the verb *man.*

5 The parser could call on the general knowledge component to explore the discourse for any clues about the meaning of this puzzling sentence. In a discourse text like *The young fishermen all had to leave the village*, a situation in which *The old man the boats* would be a much more acceptable interpretation.

SAQ 25
Of the possible strategies (1–5) listed above, which involve syntactic processes only and which suggest an interaction with other components?
(*Hint*: Strategies which analyse sentences in terms of alternative transitions are categorized as being within the syntactic component.)

Transition networks which allow look ahead or back-up are called **augmented transition networks (ATNs)**. This is because they have the 'augmented' facility to suspend judgement about a group of words by holding them in a temporary store called a **register** while they look ahead or consult other transitions as necessary. Registers allow parsers to take context into account before deciding which transitions to follow in the syntactic networks shown in Figure 2.4.

Marcus (1980) developed a computer parser called **PARSIFAL**. He proposed that a program will not simulate human parsing successfully if it carries forward all alternative hypotheses about possible structures or if it backtracks and starts parsing again from scratch. Instead, he claims that a parser program must follow three principles:

1 It must be responsive to word-by-word input, but;
2 It should reflect expectations derived from the partially constructed syntactic structures, and;
3 It can look ahead to a limited extent.

It is (2) and (3) which free the parser from relying only on the words already input, although the prohibition on backtracking means that errors cannot be corrected. In fact, it is claimed that PARSIFAL makes the same errors as a human when faced with a 'garden path' sentence. The analysis of *The old man* as an NP followed by puzzlement at *the boats* is a typical example of a garden path sentence. These are called **garden path sentences** because they lead the listener up the garden path before he or she realizes the appropriate meaning. Milne (1982) gives some examples of the kinds of garden path sentences by which PARSIFAL is fooled just as human language understanders would be by failing to look ahead far enough to decide between possible syntactic structures. A typical sentence is *The shooting of the prince shocked his wife because she thought he was an excellent marksman* (originally reported in Foss and Hawkes, 1978).

SAQ 26
In the 'shooting of the prince' sentence, write down the likely 'garden path' inter-pretation of the first words of the sentence and the subsequent interpretation of the sentence meaning of the whole sentence:
(a) Who is doing the shooting?
(b) Who is being shot?
(c) What shocked his wife?

Another technique for investigating garden path sentences was devised by Crain and Steedman (1985) to test the hypothesis that semantic plausibility can affect the syntactic difficulty of parsing a garden path sentence. They asked subjects to judge whether sentences were gram-matical or not (see Section 3.1). They compared sentences like *The teachers taught by the Berlitz method passed the test* and *The children taught by the Berlitz method passed the test*. Subjects judged the first sentence as being ungrammatical more often than the second sentence. Crain and Steedman's explanation was that in the first sentence the words were interpreted as indicating that the teachers used the Berlitz method to teach. The second sentence was more often judged as a grammatical sentence because it was more plausible to assume that the children were being taught by the Berlitz method.

As you will have gathered, garden path sentences are often quoted in psycholinguistics because they provide a good test of whether a computer program, or indeed a human, can cope with them. But in normal discourse speakers and writers intend their language to be immediately understandable and so they do everything possible to avoid potentially ambiguous sentences. Clark and Murphy (1982) refer to a principle of **audience design**. By this they mean that language users give their audience all the necessary clues needed to avoid ambiguity and confusions such as those responsible for garden path sentences. However, sometimes things go wrong in spite of all our best efforts. An amusing example is quoted by Parsons (1969): *Completing an impres-sive ceremony, the Admiral's lovely daughter smashed a bottle over her stern as she slid gracefully down the slipways.* Because of our tendency to make inferences about the situation being described, the writer — and probably many of his readers — simply didn't notice the ambiguity of the possible references for the pronouns 'her' and 'she'.

Examples like this seem to indicate that general knowledge about the relative plausibility of sentences does have an influence on how those sentences are understood. Let us explore further the idea that, however good the back-up and look ahead facilities of a syntactic parser, perhaps the most effective strategy is to allow interaction with seman-tic processing and general knowledge in order to resolve potential am-biguities. The next section describes a computer model which operates in this way.

3.4   Winograd's interactive model of language understanding

A classic example of a modular model of language understanding was Winograd's **SHRDLU computer program**, which caused a tremendous stir in 1972 as an early attempt to introduce different types of knowledge into a computer program dealing with language. Winograd's (1972) model was modular because it proposed separate modules for syntax, semantics and world knowledge. However, it was also an interactive model because it was possible for the modules to call up information from other modules when necessary to contribute to the final interpretation of a sentence.

All the input sentences were concerned with instructions for moving different types of blocks around in a blocks world displayed as on a computer screen (see Figure 2.5). The blocks can be 'moved around' by a pointer which can change the position of the blocks on the screen.

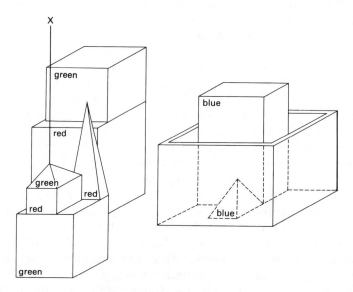

Figure 2.5   SHRDLU: blocks world (adapted from Winograd, 1972)

Figure 2.6 shows the three modules incorporated in the SHRDLU program. The Syntax Module contains syntactic rules formulated as augmented transition networks. The Semantics Module contains a lexicon and semantic selection rules for building up semantic representations, and the Blocks Module contains general knowledge about the position of the blocks at any one time (i.e. world knowledge limited to the tiny world of a small number of blocks on a screen).

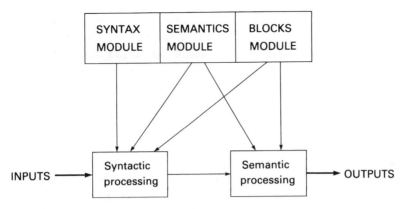

Figure 2.6   SHRDLU modules

Winograd argues that the modules must be able to pass information to each other when required. You can see the need to consult different modules by considering the command *Put the green pyramid on the block in the box.* In terms of a purely syntactic analysis, there are two possible ways to group the noun phrases in the sentence, as indicated by the positioning of the brackets:

1 *Put (the green pyramid) on (the block in the box)*, i.e. move the green pyramid and place it on top of a block which is already in the box.
2 *Put (the green pyramid on the block) in (the box)*, i.e. move the green pyramid, which is now on top of a block, and put it on the floor of the box.

SAQ 27
Using brackets, as in the above example, write down two possible syntactic analyses for the sentence *John went down the road in a bus.* Why is only one interpretation likely to be taken seriously?

To deal with a potentially ambiguous sentence like *Put the green pyramid on the block in the box*, the Syntax Module in Winograd's program is able to call on the Semantics Module and the Blocks Module to settle which of the two possible syntactic analyses is correct. For instance, the Semantics module would confirm that the verb *put* combined with names of two blocks can be constructed as a meaningful sentence involving putting one block on another block. At this point, reference would be made to the Blocks Module. Referring to its knowledge of where all the blocks are (as shown in Figure 2.5), it would report that either interpretation is possible because a green pyramid is currently on a red block and so could be moved from there to the floor of the box; equally, the green pyramid could be placed on top of the blue block which is already in the box.

While the Syntax Module is attempting to build up a syntactic structure for a sentence, it can call in the Semantics and Blocks Modules in order to resolve potential ambiguities. Thus, rather than relying solely on syntactic back-up and look forward procedures, interaction with semantic processing (and indeed also with knowledge of the Blocks world) is possible in order to short-circuit semantic interpretations. Winograd's computer model is a **heterarchical model**. In contrast to strictly hierarchical models, Winograd's program has some of the characteristics of independent processing modules and some of the characteristics of an interactive model. The most important characteristic of a heterarchical model is that processing can be interrupted in order to consult other processing modules. In later versions of Winograd's theory there was an even greater emphasis on the need to understand the discourse in which individual sentences are embedded (Winograd, 1980; Winograd and Flores, 1986).

To sum up the conclusions of this section, the cross-modal priming experiments provide evidence of independent processing. On the other hand, attempts to write computer programs incorporating syntactic parsers has led in the direction of interaction between modules. These contrasts will be discussed further in Section 5.

Summary of Section 3

- The ability to make grammatical judgements, ignoring the meaning of sentences, is evidence for syntax as an independent processing component.
- Cross-modal priming experiments show that, when processing is on-line, availability of lexical items occurs independently of syntactic structure of a sentence context. It is only after syntactic processing is complete that either a verb or a noun is selected as an appropriate lexical category.
- Many computer models include a syntactic parser for analysing the syntactic structures of sentences. Augmented transition networks operate by following transitions to identify the syntactic components of a sentence.
- When there are alternative syntactic constructions, computer programs like PARSIFAL use limited look ahead procedures, which can be compared with those used by humans, especially when dealing with garden path sentences.
- One strategy is to allow the syntactic parser to refer to the semantic processing of a sentence is order to decide between alternative syntactic structures. Winograd's classic SHRDLU program (1972) is a well-known computer model in which the Syntax Module calls on semantic rules and general knowledge of the world when building up an understanding of sentence structures.

4   Discourse processing and general knowledge

The point was strongly made in Part I, Section 5, that sentences rarely occur in isolation — except when quoted in books about language! Sentences are strung together to make up coherent texts. Understanding a text or discourse is more than simply understanding each sentence as it comes along. Readers are constantly making inferences to aid their understanding of the macrostructure of a text. Processing at this level involves interpretative processing which takes into account the macrostructure representation that is being built up for the whole text. The meaning allotted to each sentence will depend on the knowledge that is being built up in the mind of the reader. The contrast here is between the representations of individual sentences (linguistic processing) and the interpretations of texts (discourse processing).

One distinction which can be made is between the types of inferences that are necessary at different levels of understanding. In order to build up a representation of a sentence, **necessary inferences** have to be made, for instance, about the components of a noun phrase or the selection restrictions for combining word meanings. These necessary inferences are part of purely linguistic processing.

At the level of discourse, all sorts of other kinds of inferences are available. These are usually termed **elaborative inferences** because they go beyond the actual text. In Part I, Section 5, many examples were given of bridging inferences which bridge gaps between statements in order to infer meanings. These are a type of elaborative inference because they are not strictly necessary for constructing linguistic representations for individual sentences. Rather, they help to elaborate the full interpretation of a whole discourse. Language understanding in its widest sense depends on inferences which draw on social, situational and discourse expectations. Relying on probable meanings and expectations provides a short-cut to correct interpretations of potentially ambiguous sentences. Sometimes assumptions are so strong that they can override accuracy, as in the experiment reported in Part I, Section 3.3, in which subjects assumed that it was the lifeguard who saved the bather rather than the other way round (Herriot, 1969).

It is easy enough to emphasize the importance of knowledge-based inferences, but it has not proved so easy to formulate the underlying knowledge representations in a precise way. Human knowledge processing appears to be effortless and unlimited. Yet attempts to incorporate knowledge in language understanding computer programs have been limited to small domains of knowledge, such as Winograd's toy blocks or Schank's scripts representing events like visits to restaurants.

4.1   General knowledge inferences: scripts revisited

In Part I, Section 5.2, Schank's restaurant script was presented as a representation of knowledge about expected events in a restaurant. Based on this kind of knowledge, a language processor is able to make elaborative inferences about likely events in order to make sense of texts.

Schank and his colleagues (Schank and Abelson, 1977) incorporated scripts in a computer program for understanding stories about events like visiting restaurants. Script information about roles and events was keyed into the computer. Subsequently, short 'stories' were keyed in and the computer used the information in the scripts to produce an interpretation based on inferences about the normal order of events in restaurants. The program was called **SAM,** standing for **Script Applier Mechanism**. A sample of SAM's input and output is shown below; SAM's output is shown in capital letters:

Input:
John went to a restaurant. The waiter gave John a menu. The waiter came to the table. John ordered lobster. John was served quickly. John left a large tip.

Questions and answers:
Q: What did John eat?

A: LOBSTER

Q: Who gave John the menu?

A: THE WAITER

Q: Who gave John the lobster?

A: PROBABLY THE WAITER

Q: Who paid the bill?

A: PROBABLY JOHN

Q: What happened when John went to the table?

A: JOHN SAT DOWN AND THE WAITER GAVE HIM A MENU

Q: Why did John get a menu?

A: SO HE COULD ORDER

Q: Why did John give the waiter a large tip?

A: BECAUSE HE WAS SERVED QUICKLY

Paraphrase:
JOHN WENT TO A RESTAURANT. JOHN LOOKED FOR A TABLE. JOHN WENT TO THE TABLE. JOHN SAT DOWN IN THE CHAIR. JOHN GOT THE MENU FROM THE WAITER. JOHN READ THE MENU. THE WAITER WENT TO THE TABLE. JOHN ORDERED LOBSTER. THE COOK PREPARED THE

LOBSTER. THE WAITER GOT THE LOBSTER FROM THE COOK. THE WAITER SERVED JOHN THE LOBSTER. JOHN ATE THE LOBSTER. JOHN INDICATED TO THE WAITER HE WOULD LIKE TO GET THE BILL FROM HIM. JOHN GOT THE BILL FROM THE WAITER. JOHN LEFT THE WAITER A LARGE TIP. JOHN PAID THE BILL. JOHN LEFT THE RESTAURANT.

Summary:

JOHN WENT TO A RESTAURANT AND ATE LOBSTER.

SAQ 28
List some inferences in the paraphrase which are not stated in the input story.

Despite the impressive performance of SAM in understanding simple stories about restaurants, Schank has himself pointed out some of the inadequacies of scripts as a complete explanation of the role of inferences in language and understanding. For one thing, there would have to be an enormous proliferation of scripts for all possible sequences of events: dressing in the morning, catching a bus, going on an aeroplane, buying things in a supermarket, going to the hairdresser, going to the doctor, going to the dentist and so on, and so on.

4.2   St John's story gestalt model

A more recent report of a model of knowledge-intensive processes in text comprehension (St John, 1992) refers back to the work of Schank and Abelson (1977) on representing scripts. The objectives of St John's program are similar to those of Schank's programs. Of particular interest are St John's comments about the aims of his program. It is designed to be capable of making inferences, including coherence inferences to make sense of current inputs and prediction inferences to help make sense of future inputs. **Coherence inferences** are an example of elaborative inferences. **Predictive inferences** enable a reader to formulate expectations about what is likely to happen next. The story grammars described in Part I, Section 5.1, provide examples of being able to make sense of a story by predicting likely events.

St John (1992) developed a computer model in which short texts were keyed into a computer from which it built up generalizations about what it would expect to find in certain script-like situations. It has to be admitted that the 'texts' conveyed fairly simple information. For example, the program was told that *all* expensive restaurants are far away and that the person who pays the bill *always* gives a tip. On the other hand, the size of the tip has to be inferred from the person who tips, whether that person is mean or extravagant (based on prior experience), and the quality of the restaurant (an expensive restaurant or a cheap restaurant).

The first phase for the computer program was a massive training stage in which the program was presented with the truly enormous number of one million inputs. These inputs were in the familiar form of case frames (e.g. *Albert* (Agent) *paid* (Action) *the bill* (Object)). A big set of inputs of this kind is called a **corpus**, which is the Latin word for body (i.e. a large body of data input to the program). The inputs provided information about several types of script situations, including travel as well as restaurants. From these inputs the program deduced what St John calls **story gestalts**, each of which incorporates information about a set of script events. It is on the basis of these story gestalts representing script information that the program can make inferences. This is why St John called his model a story gestalt model.

In the second phase the program was given a very brief text and asked certain questions. The questions took the form of inputting a single word like *paid* and the program had to respond with the likely Agents, Objects, Recipients and Locations. The responses gave a probability figure to each inference; for example, that Albert was (.9) likely to pay the bill and Clement was only (.1) likely to pay the bill.

Input text:
Albert and Clement decided to go to a restaurant.
The restaurant was expensive.
Clement paid the bill.

DECIDED TO GO				ORDERED		
agent:	Clement	.9		agent:	Clement	.8
	Albert	.4			Albert	.1
destination:	restaurant	.9		patient:	cheap wine	.6
					expen. wine	.1
QUALITY				**PAID**		
patient:	restaurant	.9		agent:	Clement	.9
					Albert	.1
value:	expensive	.9				
				patient:	bill	.9
DISTANCE				**TIPPED**		
patient:	restaurant	.9		agent:	Clement	.9
					Albert	.1
value:	far	.9				
				patient:	waiter	.9
				manner:	small	.4
					big	.1

Figure 2.7 Responses by the St John program (adapted from St John, 1992)

The way the program was tested is shown in Figure 2.7. At the top of Figure 2.7 is a short text input to the program in the form of three sentences which can also be represented as case frames. The first sentence can be allocated a case frame as follows:

Albert and Clement	*decided to go*	*to a restaurant*
Agents	Action	Destination

SAQ 29
Write down the appropriate case-frame analysis for *Clement paid the bill*. (Note that St John uses the case 'Patient' where others would use the 'Object' case).

The program was then tested with certain action words and had to provide probabilities for the correct fillers for the case slots. The first example of an action is DECIDED TO GO. The program responds by stating that the Agents are likely to be *Clement* (.9) and *Albert* (.4) and that the Destination is (.9) likely to be a restaurant.

Not surprisingly, given the information in the short text that *The restaurant was expensive*, when tested with the word QUALITY the program agrees that the restaurant is expensive (.9). The next test is DISTANCE. Based on its prior experience that expensive restaurants are always far away, again the program has little difficulty in making the inference that the restaurant is far (.9).

The responses to ORDERED, PAID, and TIPPED are based on prior knowledge of Albert and Clement. The program has been informed that the person who pays the bill also orders the meal and gives a tip. The third sentence in the text is *Clement paid the bill*. This allows the inferences that Clement ordered (.8), paid (.9) and tipped (.9).

SAQ 30
The size of the tip depends on:
1 tips are only paid in expensive restaurants
2 tips are paid by the person who pays the bill
3 whether a person is extravagant or mean.
(Note that the program already knows that Clement is a person who orders cheap wine.)
What explanation would you give for the program's response to the input TIPPED?

How should St John's (1992) model be evaluated? Certainly, the responses in Figure 2.7 are impressive. But then so are SAM's responses to the lobster story. One big difference is that the St John 'story gestalt' model made up its own scripts based on a million plus inputs. This is in contrast to Schank and Abelson (1977), who input the script information directly to the SAM program. This may seem a big difference in favour of the St John model. But, in order to give the story gestalt program the information it needed to make inferences, the corpus of inputs fed into the program was carefully planned so as to limit its knowledge about who is likely to order the meal and to pay the bill, just as in Schank's restaurant script.

Like Schank, St John also found it was hard for the program to know when it should switch from one script to another. For instance, if one type of car was always driven to the airport in an airport script, the program would deny that the same car could be driven to a restaurant. The difficulty is how to generalize information from one script to another, to realize that there are common actions involved in driving to different destinations or in making appointments to visit both doctors and dentists.

St John admits that the script input to SAM represents systematic information that his program would not be able to infer from its inputs. Nevertheless, the claim is that the story gestalt approach is a better representation of the way in which humans gradually accumulate information and develop inferences about the likely probabilities of events. In both cases, the aims of the computer programs are to represent general knowledge about events and to demonstrate the importance of inferences based on general knowledge in understanding discourse.

There is perhaps little disagreement that general knowledge comes into play when making sense of connected discourses, whether they are a few sentences long and about restaurants, or whether they involve understanding the whole of this book. However, a more general question concerns the feasibility of distinguishing between linguistic knowledge and general knowledge as two separate and independent modules involved in language processing.

The general conclusion from this section is that it is not an easy matter to isolate distinct modules in language processing. If you look back to the linear and interactive models in Figures 2.1 and 2.2, you will see that in the linear model general knowledge only affects the final stage of discourse processing. The lexical, syntactic and semantic processing modules represent purely linguistic processing. In Figure 2.2, the same modules are responsible for linguistic processing. However, the arrows allow for interaction between modules and for all types of knowledge to be available at every stage.

Summary of Section 4

- A distinction can be drawn between necessary inferences required for linguistic processing and elaborative inferences required for discourse processing.
- Discourse processing involves elaborative and bridging inferences based on general knowledge in order to build up a macrostructure interpretation of a whole discourse or text.

- General knowledge has been incorporated in computer programs as scripts representing knowledge of situations and events (Schank and Abelson, 1977, and St John, 1992). The aim is to enable the programs to make elaborative and predictive inferences which demonstrate understanding of brief texts.

5   *Concluding issues*

The main theme of Part II has been a contrast between two models. One model assumes that each linguistic process takes place independently and has to be completed before the next process can begin. This was described as a linear model (see Figure 2.1). The other model assumes that linguistic processes are not independent, so that different types of linguistic information can be taken into account in language understanding. This was described as an interactive model (see Figure 2.2).

Theoretical arguments have been put forward claiming that one or other model is more 'cognitively efficient' in aiding rapid language understanding. One claim is that self-contained specialist modules can rapidly recognize words, assess word meanings or analyse the syntactic structure of a sentence. The counter-argument is that it is more economical to bring in as many types of linguistic information and general knowledge as required to sort out ambiguous sentences. Cross-modal priming experiments are designed to investigate on-line processing when people are actually processing sentences. Evidence from priming experiments has demonstrated that, during ongoing processing of sentences, the lexical, syntactic and semantic modules operate independently. While all these processes are presumably occurring at the same time, lexical access is not influenced by the syntactic or semantic structure of a sentence. These results are evidence for the independence of modules, as in the linear model.

There are some methodological comments which can be made about these cross-modal priming experiments. First, the time intervals are very small. After only 200 milliseconds (a fifth of a second), the syntactic and semantic structure of a sentence do have a priming effect on selecting appropriate lexical meanings, showing that interaction is occurring. So, if the modules are only independent for such a very brief time, is it reasonable to conclude that the linear model of language processing is correct?

Another question which can be asked is whether the tasks involved in priming experiments approximate to realistic language understanding processes. How often is it that language users see words flashed very briefly on a computer screen and are asked to name the word or, perhaps even more bizarrely, decide whether a string of letters is a word (the lexical decision task)? Rather than tapping natural language processing, such experiments may be testing subjects' ability to perform peculiar tasks set by psychologists. The experiments are robust in the sense that people act in predictable ways in certain specific circumstances, but this is not necessarily what happens in normal language understanding.

In contrast to the results of the priming experiments, computer models have included facilities for interactive processing. Cottrell's model incorporated the simultaneous activation of lexical case slots, words and word senses in order to select appropriate sentence meanings. Winograd's model included a facility for a syntactic module to refer to semantic and general knowledge modules as required.

Computer programs which aim to model the interpretation of sentences in discourse have incorporated general knowledge, often in the form of script representations of situations and events. Schank and Abelson (1977) and St John (1992) are examples. These programs are intended to provide the type of information required for making the kinds of elaborative inferences necessary to build up a macrostructure of a whole text. However, computer models are also vulnerable to methodological criticisms. It can be argued that such programs work by completely different procedures from those employed by human language understanders. It is certainly true that the rules and knowledge incorporated in programs are extremely simple and that consequently they can deal with only a tiny set of sentences about a tiny knowledge domain.

It will never be possible to convince computer modellers that anything can be learned from the most careful psycholinguistic experiments. Equally, experimenters are unlikely to accept that computer models have the advantage of having to specify precise rules which can be tested against their ability to simulate some aspects of language understanding.

The implications of the experiments described in Technique Boxes and the computer models in relation to the linear and interactive models are summarized in Table 2.1.

It might be concluded from the discussion of the role of general knowledge in Section 4 that it is genuinely impossible to distinguish between linguistic knowledge and general knowledge. What does seem indisputable is that language users bring to language processing a conceptual apparatus of knowledge, expecting language to conform to what is known about the world, such as that birds fly, cows eat grass, and people throw balls.

Table 2.1   Evidence for two models of language processing

Linear independent model	Interactive model
• On-line semantic priming experiments	• Cottrell's lexically-based model for semantic analysis
• Grammatical judgements (regardless of meaning)	• Winograd's program model calling up information from other modules
• On-line syntactic priming experiments	• Role of general knowledge in Schank's and St John's knowledge-based computer programs

The question is whether there are specifically linguistic processes which define a language user's ability to speak a language. Certainly, we all know what it is like *not* to have the linguistic competence necessary to speak a particular language. If we have no knowledge of the vocabulary of a language, we have no lexicon to be accessed. If we know a few words but are totally unaware of the grammar, efforts at communication are pitiful indeed. One way of thinking about the task of learning a language is that language learners have to map the vocabulary (lexicon), grammar (syntax) and rules for building up sentence meanings (semantics) on to their prior knowledge of the world. One reason why learning a new language is so difficult is because each language uses slightly different patterns of word meanings in the lexicon and different syntactic rules to express subtle differences in mapping reality.

Further reading

As for Part I, Garnham's book *Psycholinguistics: Central Topics* (1985) is an excellent source for many of the topics and experiments discussed in Part II.

Winograd's computer program, Schank's script-based model and other similar models are described in Greene (1986) *Language Understanding: A Cognitive Approach.*

Cottrell's lexically-based model is described in his book *A Connectionist Approach to Word Disambiguation* (1989). This is quite a difficult book, but the last two chapters give an interesting historical account of computer programs for understanding language.

Finally, a book by Steven Pinker, *The Language Instinct* (1994), is a fascinating read and tackles the issue of the extent to which linguistic abilities are inbuilt into the human brain.

Part III
Anaphoric Reference

Mark Coulson

Contents

1   Introduction   93
1.1   What is anaphoric reference?   93
1.2   Why study anaphors?   93
1.3   Some terminology   97

2   Types of anaphor   98
2.1   Pro-anaphors   99
2.2   Noun phrase anaphors   100
2.3   Ellipsis   101
2.4   Deixis, sense and reference   103

3   Processing anaphors   105
3.1   Two models of anaphoric processing   105
3.2   The time-course of information use   107
3.3   Finding antecedents: the rules of resolution   110
3.4   Lexical information and non-linguistic information   113
3.5   Breaking the rules   116
3.6   Returning to the models   118

4   Placing anaphors in context   119
4.1   Focus   119
4.2   Sentential focus   121
4.3   Discourse focus   123
4.4   Anaphor antecedent distance   127
4.5   Intonation   129

5   The bonding process   131
5.1   The final interpretation   131
5.2   The immediacy of resolution and anaphoric ambiguity   132
5.3   Anaphors and inferences   135

6   Conclusions   136

1   *Introduction*

Part III presents an in-depth look at a particular area of language understanding known as anaphoric reference. It attempts to demonstrate both how important an understanding of anaphoric reference is, and how studying it can tell us a great deal about the rest of the cognitive system responsible for processing language.

1.1   *What is anaphoric reference?*

In Part I of one of the companion volume in this series, *Problem Solving: Current Issues* (Kahney, 1993), an example of a 'typical' problem was 'What does "anaphoric" mean?' An answer can now be provided! **Anaphors** in general are *words or phrases which relate new information to ideas or objects that have been mentioned previously*. In Greek, anaphora literally means 'carrying back'. In the three sentences below, the underlined anaphors serve to indicate exactly who it was that bought the beer. We will adopt the convention of underlining the anaphor of interest throughout the remainder of Part III:

> Mark and Ana went to the shops where <u>they</u> bought some beer.
> Mark and Ana went to the shops where <u>she</u> bought some beer.
> Mark and Ana went to the shops where <u>he</u> bought some beer.

In order to understand who it was that bought the beer, we have to link (or 'carry back') the anaphor, which in the examples above is a pronoun, to one or more of the entities that have already been introduced in the discourse. This process is termed **anaphoric reference**.

Pronouns such as *he, she* and *they* are by far the most common type of anaphor in English. Not only this, they are also the most researched and well-understood of the anaphors. As a result, although this part is about anaphors in general, a lot of what will be said is concerned with pronouns. Section 2 will describe the main types of anaphor.

1.2   *Why study anaphors?*

Why are anaphors important in language? When we ask a question about the use of anaphors we inevitably introduce all sorts of other questions about the nature of language and how it is represented and processed. If we are to provide a model of how language is processed, these fundamental aspects have to be addressed. The study of anaphoric processing can often throw light on some of the broader issues that have been raised in Parts I and II.

Take the following story as an example (example sentences in Part III are numbered sequentially as an aid to identification):

> (1) Ana was going on holiday with Mark and Simon. (2) She was going to lie on the beach doing nothing for two weeks. (3) Mark had been in charge of all the arrangements, he had booked them a flight that left at four in the afternoon. (4) When they got to the airport a stewardess told them that fog was delaying the departure of their plane. (5) After a long wait they finally boarded the plane. (6) Ana was first up the steps where the pilot was waiting to meet them.
> (7) 'Hello', she said, 'I hope we manage to take off in all this fog.'
> (8) 'I'm sure there'll be no problem', came the reply.

This discourse is quite unproblematic and easy to understand. However, many of the anaphors contained within it are potentially ambiguous and require some degree of processing before they can be linked with the correct entity. The nature of this processing and the different sources of information which have to be considered when attempting anaphoric resolution are outlined below. Incidentally, to emphasize just how common anaphors are, the story above contains at least ten examples. By the time you have read to the end of this part you should be able to identify the majority of them.

SAQ 31
Try to identify as many of the anaphors in the story above as you can.

Using linguistic information to resolve anaphors
How do we know that 'she' in sentence (2) refers to Ana, and not to Mark or Simon? The processor which works out who the anaphor refers to must have access to information about gender which informs it that Ana is female whereas Mark and Simon are both male, and furthermore that 'she' can only refer to a female. A less straightforward decision is made in sentence (7), where 'she' could plausibly refer to either Ana, the pilot, or the stewardess. However, the decision that 'she' is Ana seems just as automatic as in (2).

The distinction between Ana and 'the pilot' is that whilst Ana carries a **linguistic marker** (the word can only refer to a female), the pilot does not. Pilots are probably more likely to be male, although of course they do not have to be. There is nothing linguistically problematic about a pilot who is a 'she'.

Given that gender is not always directly specified by the nature of the word itself, we need to know how knowledge of gender is represented and accessed in order to understand how pronouns are processed. In order to do this, we have to look at the way in which information is represented by the listener/reader. On hearing or reading 'the pilot', do we assume a particular gender or is this left open until more information becomes available?

Immediacy of processing

We seem to understand the anaphors in the story as soon as we read them. Anaphoric resolution therefore seems to be an *immediate* (on-line) process. This may be a feature of well-structured, unambiguous prose. Where there *are* ambiguities, it might be sensible for the language processor to delay resolution. In (9) below, for example, do we immediately make a 'best guess' as to what the pronoun refers to, or do we wait until further information arrives?

(9) Mark was driving his new Mercedes. <u>It</u> was a beautiful . . .
   . . . car.
   . . . day.

There would seem to be two options. Either the anaphor can be immediately resolved along the lines of the 'best guess', or the language processor can wait for further information to become available before making its decision. Obviously, both strategies have their advantages and disadvantages. The immediate process frees the language understanding system from having to keep an anaphor in working memory, but achieves this at the risk of making mistakes. The delayed process does not make mistakes, but makes additional and perhaps unacceptable demands on working memory. Remember that, as in Part II, 'the language processor' means the cognitive mechanism which carries out language processing.

Using non-linguistic knowledge to resolve anaphors

Referring again to the pilot in the story, if we are biased towards thinking of pilots as male, then this knowledge must be based on our knowledge of the world rather than our knowledge of English. The inference 'pilot is male' is therefore based on *non-linguistic* information. There is nothing inherent in the *word* that labels a pilot as male (unlike, for example, fire*man*); rather, it is something that rests on our knowledge of the *world* and the pilots which exist in it. If the pilot–male inference is made immediately, this would imply that the processor has immediate access to non-linguistic information, and thus that the processing system should be characterized as interactive rather than linear. Remember that one of the essential features of the interactive model described in Part II is that the results of inferences based on real-world knowledge are available to guide the interpretation of language.

Focus

How do we know the pronoun in sentence (3) refers to Mark and not Simon? Mark is at the forefront of the story at this point, as the sentence concerns something he has done (booking the flight). We seem to infer automatically that any reference must be to him. This general phenomenon is known as **focus**. Focus is also a non-linguistic source of information. It helps us to understand what might otherwise be ambiguous. Although both Mark and Simon can be referred to using 'he', only Mark is being held in working memory at the time the pronoun is encountered, and so only Mark is available for the pronoun to link to. Anaphoric reference is therefore very dependent on the contents of working memory.

A stronger example of focus can be found in sentence (7), where 'she' could refer to either Ana, the pilot, or the stewardess. Here, it seems to be a general focusing process operating at the story level which causes us to prefer 'she' as referring to Ana. The stewardess and the pilot are only subsidiary characters whereas Ana is the subject of the whole story, and the pronoun prefers to link with the focus of the story. In order to understand anaphoric reference, we need to understand how focus works at both the level of the sentence and the story (or, more generally, the discourse).

Activity 1
Still not convinced that anaphoric reference is important in language understanding? Try rewriting the short story on p.94, replacing pronouns with names or titles. Does it make it easier or harder to understand?

All the sources of information outlined above make greater or lesser contributions to anaphoric resolution. Although numerous, it will prove useful to consider two general types of information: linguistic information which concerns syntax, gender and number and lexical meaning, and non-linguistic information which includes focus and scripts (and more specific world knowledge such as cultural views of gender).

Scripts as sources of antecedents
One of the dangers of looking at anaphoric processing (and in fact most cognitive processes) is that it all seems so rapid and natural that to suggest there may be a problem seems ridiculous. However, with a little thought it can be seen that resolution often involves a great deal of inferencing. As in many psychology textbooks, a good starting point is in a restaurant:

> (10) Mark and the waiter argued for a long time about the food. In the end <u>he</u> was so disgusted that <u>he</u> got up and left.

The pronoun is ambiguous in as much as it could refer either to Mark or the waiter. The two 'he's' could even refer to different people. The fact that we have little difficulty in deciding to whom both 'he's' refer implies that we are drawing an inference about who is likely to be leaving a restaurant in disgust. Where does this knowledge come from? It is obviously something to do with how scenarios in the world are typically structured. In other words, anaphoric resolution makes use of *script-based* information (Schank and Abelson, 1977 — see Part I, Section 5.2). Scripts are another kind of non-linguistic knowledge used in resolving anaphors.

1.3   Some terminology

Before going any further, it is a necessary evil that we establish a working vocabulary which can be used to refer to some of the terms discussed in the remainder of this part.

The idea, object or person to which an anaphor relates is known as the **co-referent**, or **antecedent** of the anaphor, and the two are said to **co-refer**. This means they both refer to the same object in the world (e.g. the object referred to by the name 'Mark', or 'Ana', etc.). We say that anaphors co-refer rather than refer because there is always an indirect link between the anaphor and the object it indicates. The word 'Mark' refers to an object in the world, and 'he' can be used to refer to the same thing when linked to 'Mark'. 'He' on its own does not refer to anything, hence it can only ever *co*-refer with an antecedent.

The process by which anaphor and antecedent are interpreted as co-referents is known as **resolution**. The **resolution processor** is also called the **co-reference processor**. The process of resolution links an anaphor to its correct co-referent, thereby accessing the antecedent's meaning. It is important to realize that the resolution processor is part of the language processor which, in turn, is part of the cognitive system, and as such resides inside your head. Information in the form of words enters this system, whether through the visual or the auditory sensory system, and is analysed for its meaning. The resolution of anaphors is simply one aspect of this overall process.

SAQ 32
Identify the anaphors and co-referents/antecedents in the following sentences, making sure you know which is which.
(a) The police took the burglar to the house he had robbed.
(b) After five years, Mark recognized Suzy the second she entered the room.
(c) When Ana saw the dog, she was amazed at how thin it was.

In addition to acting as the 'glue' which holds sentences and discourses together in meaningful wholes, anaphors are a useful way of reducing the complexity of language. Rather than forcing us to repeat names, descriptions or events, anaphors enable us to refer to them with simple labels such as 'he', 'it', 'the situation' and an infinite number of others.

Although the existence of anaphors has almost certainly arisen from a necessity to keep language as simple as possible, the fact that many types of anaphor, such as pronouns, are so general and powerful means that their processing is not always as straightforward as one might hope. As will become clear, processing an anaphor frequently entails a great deal more than just linking two words together. As relevant information can be drawn from almost anywhere, anaphoric resolution often makes use of all the processes and forms of inference that were discussed in Part II. As well as introducing a new topic in depth, this part will therefore also serve to revise some of the material presented in the rest of the book.

Summary of Section 1

- Anaphors are words or phases which link current to past information.
- Understanding how anaphors work involves taking into account many other aspects of linguistic and non-linguistic processing. These include: syntax, number, gender, lexical meaning (linguistic information); and focus, scripts and world knowledge (non-linguistic information).
- The concepts to which anaphors link are called antecedents or co-referents. Anaphors and antecedents co-refer with the same thing 'out there' in the world.
- The process by which anaphor and antecedent are linked is called *resolution* or *co-reference*.
- The availability of antecedents can be determined by what is contained in working memory at the time the anaphor is encountered.

2   *Types of anaphor*

Now that we have sketched out the bare bones of the subject, it is useful to put some meat on them and identify some of the common types of anaphor that occur. It is important to stress that what follows is not intended to be an exhaustive account of the many different types of anaphor. Nor is it intended to present details about the ways in which they are processed, which is the domain of Section 3.

One further point which should be mentioned at an early stage is that anaphors have been studied in depth by both psychologists and linguists. There is a slight difference in the way the two conceive of 'data'. For psychologists, data are the results, usually in the form of reaction times, gathered from experimental investigations. We shall consider numerous examples in the text that follows. Linguists, on the other hand, consider any normal speech act as constituting valid data, with the result that many linguistic theories are founded on examples of sentences with which fluent speakers of a language are comfortable. There is a slight problem with this interpretation, in that what may be comfortable to one person may not be to another. Where this consideration becomes important, it will be raised. Generally, though, this part will focus upon a mixture of both psychological (experimental) and linguistic (naturally occurring) data.

The main types of anaphor that will be described in this section are pro-anaphors, noun phrase anaphors, ellipsis and deixis. The distinction between them is that the first two consist of either a word or a phrase, whereas ellipsis and deixis are the result of some form of omission or absence of a word or phrase. All four types of anaphor play an important part in language understanding.

2.1   Pro-anaphors

Pro-anaphors use single words or short phrases to stand for their antecedents. There are a number of specific ways in which this can occur.

Pronouns
The simplest types of pro-anaphors are the **pronouns**. These include the personal subject pronouns (e.g. *he, she, they* and *it*), the possessive pronouns (e.g. *his, her, their* and *its*), the reflexives (e.g. *himself, herself, themselves*), the relatives (e.g. *who, which*), and many others.

The personal pronouns are useful tools for research because they can be described along three dimensions. These are syntactic case (the syntactic position of a word in a sentence), number (singular or plural), and gender (masculine, feminine, or unspecified, as with 'it'). These three constraints determine whether a particular antecedent can co-refer with a pronoun. For instance, (11), (12) and (13) are unacceptable for reasons of syntax, gender and number respectively:

(11) Ana loves <u>she</u>.
(12) The man went to the shops where <u>she</u> bought some eggs.
(13) The woman dropped <u>their</u> handbag.

SAQ 33
Sentences (12) and (13) can be placed in contexts which would make them acceptable. Indeed, the only restrictions that can be made to apply regardless of context are those arising from syntactic principles. Other inconsistencies can always be resolved by the presence of an antecedent from outside the sentence. Can you think of preceding sentences which would make (12) and (13) acceptable?

Pro-sentences

A **pro-sentence** replaces a whole sentence with words like 'such' or a sentential 'it'. Notice that, whereas pronouns typically replace only a single word, pro-sentence anaphors replace entire sentences. The 'it' at the start of the second sentence below co-refers with the entire first sentence:

> (14) Mark never learns from his mistakes. <u>It</u> is a terrible shame.

In example (14), the 'it' replaces 'Mark never learns from his mistakes'. Interestingly, pro-sentence anaphors aren't limited to referring to just one sentence. In the case below, the anaphor 'such' can co-refer with a wide variety of possible states which may require several sentences' worth of explanation:

> (15) <u>Such</u> were the contents of my mind after studying anaphoric processing.

Clearly, it is not at all obvious what the correct antecedent is in this sentence.

Pro-verbs

Not to be confused with proverbs, **pro-verbs** use forms of 'to do' to replace an action (specified by a verb) which must be detailed elsewhere. Again there is a contrast with pronouns. Pronouns replace nouns (objects). Pro-verbs on the other hand act as substitutes for verbs (actions):

> (16) Ana steals from the fridge at night. Mark <u>does too</u>, only more discreetly.

Again, pro-verbs are not restricted to co-referring with a single action:

> (17) Ana drinks like a fish and swears like a trooper. Mark <u>does too</u>, but not at the same time.

To summarize, pro-anaphors use simple words or short phrases to co-refer with persons, objects, actions, feelings and events. Although unimpressive to look at, they serve an extremely important role in language, reducing the amount of information which has to be written or spoken.

2.2   Noun phrase anaphors

Noun phrase anaphors take the form of sets of words, or phrases, which refer back to previously mentioned antecedents. They differ from pro-anaphors in that they take the form of complete noun phrases which can have meaning divorced from their antecedent. Obviously, 'he' has no meaning on its own — it is a purely co-referential term. 'The man' (a noun phrase anaphor), on the other hand, does contain some semantic information.

The two most common examples are *repeated name* anaphors (18) and *definite noun phrase* anaphors (19):

(18) Mark went for a drive and got hopelessly lost. That's <u>Mark</u> for you.

(19) Ana never lets you get a word in edgeways. <u>The woman</u> cannot stop talking.

It isn't clear whether a definite noun phrase anaphor makes sense without an antecedent:

(20) <u>That woman</u> has been criticizing the government again.

The above example suggests that, although anaphors must always find an antecedent (who 'that woman' is), these do not necessarily have to be located in the words which make up the sentence or discourse. Further examples of this type of anaphor are discussed in Section 2.4.

2.3   Ellipsis

An **ellipsis** is an invisible anaphor — at first glance it doesn't appear to be there because it is not represented by a word or phrase. Of course, since one of the advantages of anaphors is that they reduce the amount of information that has to be presented, ellipsis may be the most sophisticated of all anaphors.

Simply put, ellipsis is the result of a deletion process whereby a word or set of words (usually a verb phrase) is removed from a sentence with the resultant 'gap' acting as a signal that an antecedent is required to fill in the meaning. The most common form of ellipsis, **verb phrase ellipsis (VPE)** is the removal of a verb phrase which leaves an invisible signal behind. We shall use the symbol $\emptyset$, which is the mathematical symbol for an empty set, to identify ellipsis:

(21) I've never been to Venice but my brother has $\emptyset$, and he says it was horrible. ($\emptyset$ = 'been to Venice')

SAQ 34
Identify where the ellipsis occurs in the following, and find the antecedent:
  Are you going to the concert? Yes, I am.

The important thing about VPE is that the deleted information must retain a high degree of similarity to the antecedent. Technically, there needs to be *syntactic parallelism* between anaphor and antecedent. Because of this constraint, the meaning of an elliptical construction is dependent on the syntax of the clause which acts as the antecedent. As a result of this, we can produce examples where, although the antecedent does not differ in meaning, it does differ in structure, and when used elliptically can alter the meaning of the anaphor. An example (adapted from Garnham and Oakhill, 1989) is given below:

(22) Mark had seduced Ana. Hilary had ø, too.
(23) Ana had been seduced by Mark. Hilary had ø, too.

Notice that the elliptical sentence is identical in both examples ('Hilary had, too'). Note also that the *meaning* of the first sentence is the same in both cases. All that has changed is that in (23) the first sentence has undergone a passive transformation. This has the effect of forcing the ellipsis to co-refer with 'been seduced by Mark', as opposed to 'seduced Ana' in (22). Therefore, in (22) Hilary seduced Ana, whilst in (23) Mark seduced Hilary. This illustrates the importance of syntactic parallelism, as discussed above, in resolving ellipsis. The antecedent seems to be 'copied' into the anaphoric gap, translating its meaning directly.

The fact that ellipsis usually involves a direct copying from antecedent to anaphor can make for some unfortunate stylistic errors, as the example below indicates:

(24) I moved quickly to join the BBC's staff because I did not want anyone — least of all those working within the Corporation — to think that my commitment and dedication to the BBC were less than total, which they are.
(Letter from John Birt to *The Times*, 8 March 1993)

SAQ 35
What is wrong with the above text? Try to spot where the ellipsis occurs, and then work out what the elided material is. Compare this to what the letter was *intended* to communicate.

Although it appears that ellipsis simply involves copying an entire antecedent into a gap, it will be argued later (in Section 5.1) that the story cannot be as simple as this. To start with, small changes in things such as verb tenses do not seem to have an effect:

(25) Bill swept the floor because Sarah wouldn't ø.

The inflection of the verb has changed (ø = 'sweep the floor' in the present tense, whereas the antecedent is 'swept the floor' in the past tense). Such small changes appear to be perfectly acceptable to the language processor in dealing with this kind of construction.

One interesting and possibly important advantage of requiring syntactic parallelism is that it may help language understanding under certain circumstances. Villaume (1988) predicted that, when discourse becomes difficult to follow, there will be an increased reliance on 'formal' anaphora (e.g. VPE) which rely on structural rather than referential cues for their resolution. In plain English, when you don't understand what you are reading it's easier to keep going if the anaphors can be resolved syntactically rather than semantically. Villaume analysed a number of natural conversations, and, although the results were not significant, there was a pattern in that more difficult discourse tended to include more ellipses (which could be resolved syntactically) than easy discourse. This suggests that ellipsis may have been used as a way of making difficult discourse easier.

2.4   Deixis, sense and reference

The final kind of anaphor we will come across in this part looks like a noun phrase anaphor or pronoun but is in fact quite different and raises some interesting questions about how antecedents are located. A **deictic anaphor** co-refers with an entity that is not contained within the linguistic context — there is no word or phrase present which can act as an antecedent. Deictic pronouns are often accompanied by gestures such as pointing (returning to Greek once more, **Deixis** means 'pointing' or 'showing'). Sentence (26) contains a deictic pronoun:

(26) Look at that. (pointing towards something)

In order to be able to locate the antecedent for a deictic anaphor, we have to make use of what Lyons (1981) calls the **deictic context**. This context can include such things as gestures and visual information in addition to the actual words used (so it includes both linguistic and non-linguistic information). For example, a national newspaper (*The Independent*) has used deixis with a visual context to advertise itself:

(27) It is. Are you?

SAQ 36
As well as the deictic 'it', there are two ellipses in example (27). Can you see where they are and what their antecedents are? (Hint: they both have the same deictic antecedent).

As shown below, an anaphor can identify either the same, or a similar but not identical, entity as its co-referent:

(28) Mark made a cheese sandwich and then ate it.
(29) The man who gave his paycheck to his wife was wiser than the man who gave it to his mistress.

In (28), 'it' clearly refers to the same cheese sandwich that Mark made in the first clause. The 'it' in (29), on the other hand, must refer to another paycheck or the sentence does not make sense — if the anaphor referred to the same entity then we would have the situation of two men giving the same paycheck to two different women. (Incidentally, paycheck sentences have a long and glorious tradition in psycholinguistics and no textbook would be complete without one. The gender typing should therefore be seen in its true historical context — it in no way reflects any views of the author.)

Grinder and Postal (1971) refer to the two types of anaphor described above as **identity of reference** and **identity of sense** respectively. Identity of reference anaphors refer to exactly the same referent represented by the antecedent with which they co-refer. Identity of sense anaphors refer to a member of the same *class* of objects to which the antecedent refers. The difference between the two types of anaphor suggests that different representations may be involved in each case. The importance of identical sense versus identical reference can be seen in example (30), where the anaphor is ambiguous between the two and the sentence therefore has two possible interpretations:

(30) Ana likes her hair short, but Suzy prefers it long.

In the identical *reference* sense of 'it' (the preferred interpretation), the anaphor co-refers with the exact same antecedent (i.e. Ana's hair). This leads to the interpretation that Suzy likes Ana's hair to be long. If the pronoun is being used in an identical *sense* fashion, however, then Suzy likes *her own* hair long.

SAQ 37
As well as the identical sense and identical reference interpretations of (30) there is also a deictic version. Can you see what it is?

In short, the problem is that, although it is easy enough to understand that an anaphor is a link between what is being discussed or read at the moment and an antecedent, deixis makes it clear that locating antecedents may be problematic. Looking back at the section on ellipsis, we can also see that, whereas pronouns only need an object in the discourse to refer to ('Mark' or 'Ana' etc.), some anaphors require whole chunks of material to be copied from one place to another. Is there a unitary representation that is able to serve these diverse requirements, or can the resolution processor look in a number of different places, either sequentially or at the same time? These questions will be addressed (if not actually answered) in the remainder of this part.

Summary of Section 2

- There are four main types of anaphor: pro-anaphors, noun phrase anaphors, ellipsis, and deixis.

- Pro-anaphors are single, relatively unspecific words such as 'he', 'she', 'they' and 'it', or short phrases like 'does too'. They only have meaning in conjunction with co-referents.
- Noun phrase anaphors are more specific constructions such as 'that man', which can make sense on their own.
- Ellipses are linguistic gaps which are filled by mentally copying the antecedent from its original position into the gap.
- Deixis is where the antecedent of an anaphor is not contained within the linguistic context, forcing the reader or listener to search elsewhere, such as the deictic context or in semantic memory.
- It is not always easy to determine when an anaphor co-refers to an identical antecedent (identity of reference) or co-refers to a class of objects (identity of sense).

3   Processing anaphors

There is a vast literature concerning anaphoric processing, and it is impossible to provide anything more than a brief review here. Rather than trying to cover everything, and only providing a sketchy picture of how various anaphors are processed, this section concentrates on a number of different experiments in an attempt to answer some of the more central questions concerning anaphoric resolution.

A lot of the research we shall examine concerns pronouns. This may prompt you to retort that we are 'cheating' slightly — pronouns are the simplest form of anaphor and therefore the easiest to explain. Although we may be able to produce a neat theory of pronominal processing, our ideas may not necessarily hold true when we come to consider more complex forms of anaphor such as ellipsis. Unfortunately, even such an apparently simple endeavour as explaining how pronouns are linked to their antecedents has proved very troublesome.

3.1   Two models of anaphoric processing

Broadly speaking, there are two possible ways in which anaphors can be resolved. The two models, which we will refer to as the **single stage** and the **multi-stage** model, are outlined in Figure 3.1 overleaf.

The important differences between the two models are as follows:

1 The single stage model sees all forms of information interacting together to select one antecedent which is then linked to the anaphor. This type of model has often been called a **multiple constraint satisfaction** model, because a number of different constraints (e.g. syntax, number, focus) are all being dealt with at the same time. You

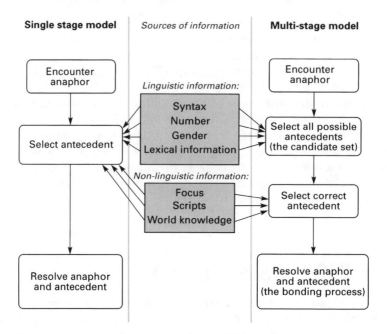

Figure 3.1   Two different models of anaphoric processing. Unshaded boxes refer to possible stages of processing, shaded boxes are different sources of information used to resolve anaphors

may notice a similarity between this model and the interactive model of language processing outlined in Part II, Section 1. There, both linguistic and non-linguistic information were allowed to interact together at all stages of processing. Indeed, in a model such as this it is not clear whether there is such thing as discrete stages of processing. Everything more or less happens at once.

In contrast to this, the multi-stage model does not see everything happening at once. Rather, the resolution of anaphor with antecedent entails a number of distinct processing stages. Each stage of processing is characterized by the types of information it makes use of. Initial processing relies solely on linguistic information, whereas later stages make use of non-linguistic sources. This model bears some similarity to the linear model of language processing with independent modules (see Part II, Section 1).

2 In the single stage model, only one possible antecedent is identified and selected. In the multi-stage model, a set of possible candidates is selected first and then the correct antecedent is selected from these at the next stage.

Having outlined two possible models, we must now look at whether they can be teased apart. As you may remember from Part II, identifying whether a processing system is independent or interactive has proved extremely difficult to do convincingly. However, there may be other means of deciding which theory offers the best explanation of anaphoric processing, and the remainder of this section is devoted to looking at some of them.

In order to be able to distinguish between the two models, we have to identify where they make different predictions about what happens to anaphors and antecedents. Once such predictions have been identified, it may be possible to design an experiment which can determine which model offers the best explanation for the data.

So where do the two models differ in their accounts of anaphoric resolution? Obviously, the single stage model views all sources of information as having their effects at the same time. It sees the interaction of these as being sufficient to produce a single antecedent which is then linked with the anaphor.

In contrast, the multi-stage model views linguistic information (syntax, number, gender and lexical information) as affecting the initial identification of possible antecedents, and the other, non-linguistic sources, such as a script for the event, as operating later on when the final selection is made. This difference in the **time-course** of information use allows us to make different predictions which can be tested experimentally.

3.2   The time-course of information use

Before we can even begin to answer the question as to which model offers the best explanation of anaphoric processing, there is one important fact that has to be taken into consideration. This fact concerns the immediacy of anaphoric resolution. If you look back at Section 1.2, it was pointed out that anaphoric resolution can be either a delayed or an immediate, on-line process. Either the anaphor is linked to its antecedent as soon as it is encountered, or resolution is delayed until more information becomes available. (Remember that this same issue about whether processes occur immediately, i.e. on-line processing, or whether they are delayed until further information becomes available, was also explored in Part II.)

If resolution is immediate, then the single stage model predicts that *all* information should become available immediately an anaphor is encountered. The multi-stage model predicts that only *linguistic* information becomes immediately available.

However, if resolution is delayed, then the models do not make different predictions which can be tested. If there is a time-lapse between

107

encountering an anaphor and resolving it, then it is not possible to decide whether resolution is a single stage process. The information may have been used at different times, but by the time the anaphor is resolved all sources will have had their effects.

Remember what was said earlier about the speed of many types of cognitive process. It may be that resolution is multi-stage, but that these stages occur extremely rapidly, and are complete by the time we can measure any effects on, for example, reading times.

The question of immediacy or delay therefore has to be addressed before we can go on to look at the time-course of information use. Techniques Boxes G and H describe experiments which have sought to answer this question.

TECHNIQUES BOX G

Immediacy versus Delay in Anaphoric Processing
(Stevenson and Vitkovitch, 1986)

Objective
To test whether pronoun assignment is made immediately or is de-layed until further information becomes available.

Method
Subjects read sentences off a computer screen and responded as to whether an ambiguous pronoun ('he' or 'she') referred to the first or the second person mentioned in the sentence. The verb following the pronoun was judged by independent judges to be either informative or uninformative as to the correct assignment. Following an informa-tive verb, the referent is unambiguous. Following an uninformative verb the referent is ambiguous.

Informative verb:
The policeman chased the thief and he *caught* him in an alley.

Uninformative verb:
The father questioned his son and he *told* him to tell the truth.

Once the verb has been encountered in the informative sentence, the pronoun assignment should be unambiguous ('he' can only be the policeman in the first sentence). The uninformative verb is unhelpful in this respect because both father and son are valid alternatives.

Results
The mean response times (in seconds) are shown below. Response time includes both reading time for the sentence and decision time to press the response button.

	Informative verb	Uninformative verb
RT	5.72	8.95

It is clear that the informative verbs speed up anaphoric resolution. Stevenson and Vitkovitch argue that, because this effect can only be due to processing occurring after the pronoun has been encountered, resolution must necessarily involve a delay. The pronoun is not being processed until after the verb has been read and comprehended.

TECHNIQUES BOX H

Immediacy versus Delay in Anaphoric Processing
(Tyler and Marslen-Wilson, 1983)

Objective
To test whether pronoun assignment is made immediately or is delayed until further information becomes available.

Method
Subjects listened to short stories over headphones and then had to articulate a probe word which appeared on a screen. Each story finished with a *continuation fragment*, which contained a pronoun. The probe word was always a pronoun which could either be an appropriate or inappropriate continuation of the story.

Example story:
As Philip was walking back from the shop, he saw an old woman trip and fall flat on her face. She seemed unable to get up again. He ran towards ... (continuation fragment)

Probe words: HER (appropriate)   HIM (inappropriate)

Results
The times taken to say the probe words (in milliseconds) are given below.

	Appropriate probe	Inappropriate probe
RT	382	432

Response times to appropriate probes were significantly quicker than those to inappropriate probes. This effect was interpreted as indicating that the pronoun in the continuation fragment had been processed immediately, and that the results of the pronoun assignment were available to affect processing of successive information.

We should be careful about generalizing the results of either experiment. The Stevenson and Vitkovitch experiment used ambiguous pronouns. Because it is impossible to identify the correct antecedent with an ambiguous pronoun, it seems obvious that the processor would wait for further information. The Tyler and Marslen-Wilson study runs into the problem that the critical pronoun in the continuation fragment ('she') had been encountered several words prior to the subject making a response. It is quite possible that the effect of the pronoun was not immediate, but rather occurred sometime during the words following.

The evidence cited above indicates that anaphoric resolution can be either virtually immediate or delayed depending on the context. It seems obvious that some references are immediately and unconsciously made whereas others may take some time. As anaphoric reference is another type of inferential process, we should not be surprised to see that it can take variable amounts of time to complete.

Because it is difficult to decide whether resolution is immediate or not, it is not possible to determine which of the two models is correct from the time-course of information use. Given that this first difference between the models is not something which can be easily tested, can we identify any further areas to investigate?

3.3   Finding antecedents: the rules of resolution

A second important difference between the two models outlined at the start of this section is the number of antecedents which can be considered as candidates for resolution. Remember that, in the single stage model, all possible sources of information are used to identify a single antecedent which is then resolved with the anaphor. There is only one stage between encountering the anaphor and selecting the correct antecedent. In the multi-stage model, any antecedent which matches the anaphor in terms of its linguistic characteristics (syntax, number, gender and lexical information) is a member of the candidate set and is carried on to a second stage of processing which uses non-linguistic information to determine which is the correct one.

The single stage model assumes that only one antecedent is activated, on the basis of information from both linguistic and non-linguistic sources. The multi-stage model allows for the possibility of multiple activation of all possible antecedents, based on linguistic information only. Therefore, a second way to investigate which model offers the best explanation of resolution is to look at what happens to potential antecedents when an anaphor is encountered. Techniques Box I describes three experiments by Janet Nicol which examine how syntax, number and gender are used to activate the antecedents of pronouns.

TECHNIQUES BOX I

Nicol's (1988) Antecedent Activation Experiments

Rationale
Nicol set out to investigate how three of the basic sources of linguistic information constraining pronominal resolution (syntax, number and gender) affect the activation levels of antecedents. She hypothesized that all three are used immediately to select possible antecedents. She also tested whether there was multiple activation of possible antecedents.

Method
All three experiments reported below used the cross-modal priming technique described in Section 2.2 of Part II. In this methodology, a subject listens to a sentence played through headphones, and at some point during the sentence a string of letters (the *probe*) is presented on a computer screen. The subject's task is to make a lexical decision — does the string of letters constitute an English word or not? For experimental sentences, the probe was either related or unrelated to the meaning of the antecedent. For instance, if the antecedent was 'fireman', a related probe could be 'ladder' and an unrelated probe could be 'larder'. The degree to which the related probe was primed relative to the unrelated probe was taken as a measure of the effect of the resolution process on antecedent activation levels. In all cases, the probe was presented *immediately* after the subject heard the pronoun in the sentence that was being presented.

Experiment 1: Syntax
Only antecedents which are syntactically compatible with the pronoun should become activated.

The landlord told the janitor that the fireman with the gas mask would protect <u>himself</u> if necessary.

The reflexive pronoun 'himself' can only co-refer with the antecedent 'fireman'. Probe words such as 'ladder' and 'alarm', which are associated with 'fireman' should therefore be primed. Probe words associated with the non-antecedent 'janitor', like 'rent' and 'brush' should not be primed.

Experiment 2: Number
Only antecedents of the correct number should be activated.

The landlord told the janitors that the fireman with the gas mask would protect <u>them</u> from getting hurt.

The plural pronoun 'them' can only co-refer with the plural antecedent 'janitors', and only words associated with this should be primed.

Experiment 3: Gender
Finally, gender information contained within the pronoun should also affect which antecedents are activated.

The ballerina told the janitor that the fireman with the gas mask would protect her *from getting hurt.*

Here, 'her' can only co-refer with 'ballerina' which is linguistically marked for female, and therefore only words associated with 'ballerina' should be primed.

Results
Results from all three experiments are summarized below. In all cases, the amount of priming, which is the difference in response times between the related and unrelated probe words in the lexical decision task, is shown. A positive number indicates priming and significant effects are shown in bold.

		Related	Unrelated probe	Priming probe
Syntax:	Antecedent	653	759	**106**
	Non-antecedent	703	708	-5
Number:	Antecedent	652	695	**43**
	Non-antecedent	688	683	-5
Gender:	Antecedent	688	728	**40**
	Non-antecedent	687	715	28

As can be seen from the table, in all cases only words associated with the antecedent were primed by the pronoun, leading Nicol to conclude that all three sources of information are being used immediately to select possible antecedents. In addition to this, Nicol argued that these sources of information are the *only* ones used to drive initial co-referential processes. She states that 'only structural information is available to restrict activation' (Nicol, 1988, p.74). 'Structural information' corresponds to what we have been calling linguistic information. Further experiments again demonstrated that the three sources of information would activate any and all antecedents with which they agreed. This was taken as clear support for the existence of multiple activation of antecedents at the linguistic stage.

These studies demonstrate that linguistic information is used *immediately* in antecedent selection, and also that all possible antecedents which agree with the syntax, number and gender of the pronoun are activated at the same time.

Whereas selection is immediate, the process of actually linking anaphor and antecedent may take some time. The evidence is very convincing that a filter-like selection process operates very rapidly to create a candidate set of potential antecedents. Something else then operates on this set at the next stage to select the correct antecedent. This final process is known as **bonding**. In many cases, the candidate set will only have a single member, and it may be true to say that one of the features of well-formed discourse is the production of single-member candidate sets. However, it is difficult to estimate just how widespread co-referential ambiguity is in normal speech. By simply matching the properties of each potential antecedent in the discourse with the properties of the anaphor, a great deal of time could be saved by the resolution processor (and as a result, comprehension may proceed more rapidly). As there are a potentially huge number of possible co-referents within a discourse, it would make sense to run a very quick check on all of them so as to discard the majority. Thus, if a listener encountered the pronoun 'she', all nouns that didn't fit the categories 'female, singular' would be rejected as candidates for co-reference. Whatever was left could then be passed on to the bonding process which may make use of other sources of information before coming to a final decision.

SAQ 38
Although it is stated above that only antecedents with the features 'female' and 'singular' would be selected to co-refer with 'she', this is probably not always true. Can you think of nouns that could co-refer with 'she' which do not possess one or other of these features?

Further support for this idea comes from linguistic studies of what has been termed **false bonding**. Sanford and Garrod (1989) argue that, as soon as a pronoun is encountered, the selection process operates to create a candidate set of potential antecedents. If more than one potential candidate is available, all will be selected along with the 'correct' antecedent, and under certain circumstances we may be fooled into linking the wrong antecedent with the anaphor, as in the following example:

(31) If the books are too difficult, don't get your knickers in a twist. Leave them in the library and go for a walk.

3.4   Lexical information and non-linguistic information

Whether syntax, gender and number are indeed the *only* sources of information which are used for activation is contentious. Section 4 outlines some of the non-linguistic influences, such as focus and scripts, which may be involved in the resolution process. However, although the multi-stage model seems correct in its assumption that resolution involves separate stages of processing, the question of whether only

113

linguistic information is available to the selection of antecedents process has not been clearly answered.

To use an example from Section 1.2, what is the gender of 'pilot'? In order to ascribe a gender label to pilot we have to make reference to non-linguistic world knowledge in the form of scripts. Other occupations, such as 'fireman', are different. 'Fireman' is *linguistically marked*; that is, the word itself carries information as to the gender of its referent (fire*man*). In order to find the gender of a fireman you only have to use lexical information. To deal with 'he's' and 'she's' that might co-refer with pilots you have to consult your world knowledge.

From the point of view of immediacy versus delay in processing, the selection process may be better off ignoring non-linguistic information and instead concentrating solely on linguistic information. Representations based on scripts take time to construct, because they involve building a **discourse model** of the text, and the information within a sentence is almost certainly not incorporated into the model until after the sentence has been fully processed. Because many antecedents are found in the same sentence as their anaphors, a process which waited to inspect the representation of the discourse model might be unacceptably inefficient. The fact that at least some anaphors are resolved immediately — or at least before the end of the sentence — suggests that the selection process may indeed be restricted in the types of information it has rapid access to.

Although these questions remain unanswered, there is some evidence that the selection process does indeed make reference to the discourse model when creating the candidate set (Coulson, 1991, Experiments 2–4). Note that, if the selection process is immediate, and *does* access the discourse model, this suggests that all forms of information, both linguistic and non-linguistic, are used in creating the candidate set, and therefore that the multi-stage model needs revising. Separate stages of processing do seem to exist, but it may be that all forms of information are available both for selection and bonding.

There is a lack of experimental evidence for the use of non-linguistic information in antecedent selection, but can we learn anything from an inspection of linguistic data (see the beginning of Section 2 for an account of the difference between experimental and linguistic data)?

Some expressions in everyday language *imply* the existence of antecedents which are not mentioned explicitly anywhere (refer to the discussion of deixis in Section 2.4). If the processor is able to make use of this implied information and use the results of *inference* to aid the selection process, this indicates that selection is not based solely on number, gender and syntax.

One example of antecedent selection which has received some attention from linguists is what are called **anaphoric islands** (Postal, 1969).

An anaphoric island is where co-reference is attempted with a *feature* of an antecedent as opposed to the antecedent in its entirety. Compare (32) and (33):

    (32) Max's parents are dead and he deeply misses <u>them</u>.
    (33) Max is an orphan and he deeply misses <u>them</u>.

Sentence (33) is an example of an anaphoric island. Here, 'them' refers to a feature of 'orphan' because a feature of being an orphan is that you have no parents. The lexical meaning of 'orphan' *implies*, but does not state explicitly, that Max has no parents. In order to understand this sentence some form of inference has to be drawn.

In the case of the orphan sentence, the co-reference is unacceptable, even though with some effort it can be inferred. Therefore, in this case, the processor is unable to use this lexical information in the same way as it uses syntax, number and gender. This would seem to lend support to the view that only syntax, number and gender contribute to the selection process.

However, if the implication is a little stronger, then anaphoric islands can become more acceptable. Thus, Postal argues that (34) appears quite natural whereas (35) is less so:

    (34) Mark became a guitarist because he thought <u>it</u> was a beautiful instrument.
    (35) Mark became a flautist because he thought <u>it</u> was a beautiful instrument.

Postal refers to examples (34) and (35) as *derivatives* because they contain lexical information about the features which comprise their meaning. A feature of the word 'guitarist' is a guitar, because the word refers to someone who plays the instrument. In both cases the anaphor refers to the instrument rather than the player. The reason why (34) is considered valid whilst (35) is uncomfortable is that 'guitarist' is lexically similar to 'guitar' (the correct co-referent of 'it'). The relationship between 'flautist' and 'flute' is weaker.

Incidentally, you may legitimately disagree with any or all of this. Differences in dialect (the way people actually speak) count for a lot, in anaphoric reference as much as any other aspect of language. My dialect is happy with all the examples given in this text, but if yours isn't, this section should reassure you that linguists do take these differences seriously.

Stretching the point slightly, there do seem to be examples of anaphoric islands that are perfectly acceptable. For instance, in (36) overleaf, the co-referent is the author rather than the book. We do not seem to have any difficulty interpreting it as such even if we don't know who he is:

115

(36) I just read *The Grapes of Wrath*. <u>He</u> is one of my favourite authors.

Here we are drawing on non-linguistic knowledge about books and authorship. It does seem clear from (36) that at least some examples are perfectly acceptable in normal usage. If this is so, then anaphoric islands lend additional support to the experimental evidence for the use of non-linguistic information in selection. Section 4, as already noted, also discusses the role of non-linguistic information.

3.5   Breaking the rules

So far we have largely accepted on faith (and some data) that linguistic information is capable of restricting the choice of antecedent, if not to a single case, then to a sufficiently small number that resolution is not too difficult to achieve. However, although syntax, number and gender seem to specify 'rules of selection', the processor also seems quite prepared to ignore them under certain circumstances. We need to ask, then, what other influences or sources of information license us to break the rules. Some naturally occuring examples demonstrate that rules in language are rarely, if ever, absolute.

Epicene pronouns break rules of number and gender. Examples are given below:

(37) I think I'll order a frozen Margarita. I just love <u>them</u>.
(38) You may spend a lifetime looking for the right partner. We may have already found <u>them</u>. (Dateline advertisement)

(Strictly speaking, 'epicene' only refers to violations of gender. The term is used here to refer to any pronoun which seems to 'break the rules'.)

Sentence (37) is taken from a paper by Morton Gernsbacher (Gernsbacher, 1990). Using reading time as a measure, she found that the plural pronoun was comprehended more quickly than a singular equivalent 'it'. This suggests that the epicene pronoun is preferable to a linguistically correct alternative. Notice that 'a frozen Margarita' is a singular concept, and that if the rules of number are correct it should be identified by a singular anaphor. However, as Grishman (1986) points out: 'the number ... associated with an antecedent may depend on the quantifier structure of the sentence containing the antecedent' (Grishman, 1986, p.126).

The 'quantifier structure' of a sentence is concerned with whether all the words are consistently singular or plural. The indefinite article 'a' in sentence (37) identifies the antecedent not as a single Margarita which the speaker wishes to drink, but rather the whole *class* of Margaritas. When referring to this set, which is the set of all Margaritas, it therefore makes sense to use a plural pronoun. In fact, it makes little sense to refer to one particular Margarita as being the one you love unless it had been very well mixed, in which case initial reference would undoubtedly be made with the definite article 'this'. Using a distinction raised earlier, the preferred interpretation is that of identity of sense as opposed to identity of reference (see Section 2.4).

The second example of an epicene pronoun does create a serious problem for a linguistically-based account of anaphoric resolution. The sentence pair in (38) seems intuitively valid, and yet there is a clear violation of a fundamental feature of the pronoun (although the thought may be tempting, this advert is not advocating polygamy). What distinguishes this case from (37) is that the antecedent is identified using the *definite* article (*the* right partner), and so we are left in no doubt as to the singular nature of 'them' as an anaphor. There is no obvious explanation for why 'them' is used as a singular pronoun in English, except that the language has no singular, neuter pronoun which can be used to refer to a noun like 'partner', and 'it' is considered dehumanizing. This may represent a triumph of political correctness over good grammar, or it may emphasize that language is about communication as opposed to following rules.

A related problem in English, of special interest to all scientists, concerns a situation where number is not lexically indicated. The word 'data' is actually a plural (singular *datum*). Sentences such as 'the data clearly indicates . . .' are therefore ungrammatical. Pronouns used to co-refer with 'data' should be 'they' and 'them' rather than 'it'.

With regard to the importance of syntactic information, we have already mentioned that ellipsis is heavily dependent on syntax, and that most ellipses are grammatically controlled. However, there is some evidence that we do not always apply grammatical interpretations to ellipses, and therefore that syntax is not all that important after all. Garnham and Oakhill (1987) showed that subjects tended to apply **pragmatically plausible interpretations** to ellipses rather than syntactically correct interpretations. This means they interpreted ellipses in ways which made 'real' sense as opposed to ways that followed the rules of grammar. This tendency was found to increase with increasing distance between the anaphor and its antecedent. Garnham and Oakhill argue that, although subjects *realize* they need to be looking for a syntactically parallel antecedent, the rapid decay of structural information in working memory makes searching for conceptual interpretations easier.

The fact that language is about communicating meaning, rather than adhering to rules of syntax, supports the idea that ellipsis is pragmatically rather than syntactically controlled. In fact, ungrammatical ellipses can often make a lot more sense, and communicate a great deal more, than their grammatical counterparts:

(39) 'What do Jagulars do?' asked Piglet, hoping that they wouldn't
ø.
(from *The House at Pooh Corner*, by A.A. Milne)

The exact antecedent of the ellipsis can only be guessed at, but the
context provides a clue in Piglet's previous question to Winnie the
Pooh, 'Is it One of the Fiercer Animals?' The response is a silent nod.
What Piglet is hoping Jagulars (Jaguars) don't do is fairly clear, but is
not linguistically explicit. It is clear that non-linguistic information is
contributing to the resolution of the anaphor.

3.6   Returning to the models

Can we say with any degree of confidence which of the models offers
the best explanation of anaphoric resolution? From the point of view
of answering the question of whether anaphoric resolution consists of
one or more than one stage of processing, it seems clear that there is
a two-stage selection process, with a candidate set of potential antecedents being selected before final selection of the correct antecedent and
the bonding process occur. Therefore, the multi-stage model offers a
better account of the organization of resolution.

However, this model has been shown to contain some assumptions
that may not turn out to be true. For instance, the model as it stands
sees the first stage of selection as only using linguistic information. As
Section 3.4 demonstrated, this particular assumption may prove to be
incorrect.

The universality of linguistic rules was questioned in Section 3.5. If
these rules are not always being adhered to, something must be making
the decision to ignore them. It is highly unlikely that this something is
linguistic. It is almost certainly more to do with the way in which
language is a medium of communication rather than a strictly linguistically-based system. Thus, non-linguistic information appears to be
interacting with the application of linguistic rules. So, although the
multi-stage model seems to be a good basic characterization of anaphoric
reference, there are many questions which remain unanswered.

Summary of Section 3

- Two models of anaphoric resolution were outlined — the single and
the multi-stage model.
- Determining which model offers the best explanation from the time-
course of information use was not possible because it is not clear
whether anaphoric resolution is immediate or delayed.

- The antecedents of pronouns can be specified by syntactic case, number and gender. Studies have shown how this information is used immediately.
- It has also been demonstrated that more than one antecedent can be activated in parallel — a result which supports the predictions of the multi-stage model.
- The selection process makes use of linguistic information (syntax, number and gender), including lexical information about word meanings. It may also make use of non-linguistic information (focus, scripts, world knowledge). It is not clear at what stage these different types of information exert their influence.
- Some pronouns seem to break linguistic rules, entailing varying amounts of inferencing in order to achieve successful resolution. Even an apparently grammatical phenomenon, such as ellipsis, sometimes seems to be under pragmatic, as opposed to linguistic, control.

4   Placing anaphors in context

So far, we have considered a distinction between linguistic and non-linguistic sources of information in resolution. The linguistic sources have been well characterized and described, and we have a fairly clear idea of when they are used, how rapidly they are used, and under what circumstances they are likely to be ignored.

Less has been said about how non-linguistic information has its effect. Comments about the nature of non-linguistic information have been limited to mention of 'focus' and 'scripts.' Up to now we have (deliberately) ignored the context in which anaphors are located. This section seeks to redress this imbalance, and considers how the context in which an anaphor is located affects its interpretation.

4.1   Focus

Focus was introduced in Section 1.2, where it was stated that a good rule of thumb for interpreting anaphors was to co-refer the anaphor with whatever is in current focus. So, in (40) below, the anaphor co-refers with the focus of the sentence ('the feedpipe'). Interestingly, this happens even if you don't understand what the sentence is about (Broadbent, 1973):

> (40) The feedpipe lubricates the chain, and <u>it</u> should be adjusted to leave a gap half an inch between <u>itself</u> and the sprocket.

119

But behind this simple statement lie several unanswered questions. First, and most important, what exactly do we mean by focus? Is there a way to define it and thereby predict what will be in focus at any one time? Is there only one type of focus? And what happens when the anaphor is unable to co-refer with the focused antecedent for reasons such as gender or number?

When thinking about focus it is useful to consider an analogy with spinning plates. Whenever a new concept is introduced into the discourse, a plate (the concept) is set spinning on the top of a pole. The plate which is spinning the quickest is in the focus of attention. It is the current subject of the sentence or discourse. Plates have a natural tendency to spin slower and slower (natural decay). This can be overcome by giving the plate another spin (use an anaphor). We would probably want to say that a plate once spun never completely stops turning, but is always available for a boost. This means that even concepts which have not been mentioned for a long time can still be reintroduced by using a suitable anaphor.

One side-effect of this analogy is that the faster a plate is spinning, the less you have to do to it to keep it going or make it the fastest spinning plate of all. In terms of anaphoric reference, more central concepts (faster spinning plates) require less specific anaphors (smaller boosts). Thus, focused items can be pronominalized whereas more peripheral ones may require definite noun phrase anaphors (e.g. that woman). Some support for this intuitively appealing idea comes from Fletcher (1984) who found that less specific anaphors, such as pronouns, are more likely to be perceived as co-referring with the focus of a sentence. Marslen-Wilson, Levy and Tyler (1981) also argue that full noun phrase anaphors are used to reintroduce individuals who have slipped from focus, whereas pronouns are used to maintain reference to currently focused individuals.

We should also consider whether it makes sense to talk about a single focus. Although we may have a very clear idea about what an entire chapter or book is about (such as the fact that this part is about anaphoric reference), the focus of an individual sentence may be quite different. Perhaps we need to take into account two different kinds of focus, one operating at the discourse level and one at the level of the sentence.

Hirst (1981) states that there is a **global focus**, which is what the whole discourse is about, and a **local focus**, which is what the current sentence is about. The two often coincide, but they can be at odds with one another. It is interesting to speculate on the conditions under which either global or local focus can dominate the interpretation of an otherwise ambiguous anaphor. An example is given below where the whole point of the joke is to produce a confusion between global focus, which specifies the correct co-referent, and local focus which doesn't:

(41) *Instructions for throwing a grenade:*
    Pull out the pin and throw <u>it</u>.

The antecedent specified by the global focus, which is about throwing a grenade, is the grenade itself. Therefore, the preferred co-referent of 'it' should be the grenade. However, the focus of the sentence is the pin of the grenade, and this somehow 'steals' the best-antecedent spot. The joke relies on the fact that we notice the tension between global and local focus and are aware of the stupidity of confusing the two. Crawley and Stevenson (1990) suggest that pronouns preferentially co-refer with the focus of the sentence (the local focus).

SAQ 39
The grenade sentence is actually an example of another phenomenon discussed in an earlier section. Can you remember what this phenomenon was?

Brown and Yule (1983) say the notion of focus is: 'the most frequently used, unexplained, term in the analysis of discourse' (Brown and Yule, 1983, p.70). As a rough guide to discussing focus, we shall adopt the following terminology. **Discourse focus** refers to what entire discourses are about. The discourse focus of Part III is anaphoric reference. **Sentential focus** concerns the subject of the current sentence. So the focus of this sentence is sentential focus. This distinction, as evidenced by the grenade example, is useful in determining what anaphors will prefer to co-refer with. As a first guess, it appears that sentential focus is the first place searched. As sentential focus is sometimes linguistically represented, this may also be evidence that, for pronouns at least, search begins in the linguistic representation and only if this is unsuccessful moves on to the discourse level.

Having come to a partial understanding of what we are dealing with, it is now time to look at the two types of focus in more detail.

4.2   Sentential focus

The study of sentential focus has produced a large number of different factors thought to be influential. Different experiments have suggested that the preferred antecedent is the first mentioned participant, the subject of the sentence, the antecedent closest to the anaphor, the antecedent which occupies the same syntactic position as the anaphor, the topic of the sentence, and others. One of the interesting points to be drawn from all this is that some of the factors make directly opposing predictions about which antecedent will be preferred. There is a great deal of work still to be done in this area.

Rather than embark on an examination of all of these factors, one which has been more thoroughly, and perhaps more conclusively, re-searched will be described in detail. Although this means we are un-able to gain a complete perspective on the subject, what follows should provide a taste of research into sentential focus.

Implicit causality

Grober, Beardsley and Caramazza (1978) argue that verbs carry what they term **implicit causality**. Essentially, this is a preference for assign-ing a pronoun to either the Agent or the Patient of a sentence. In the basic active sentence, the Agent is the first noun and the Patient is the second. These are referred to as NP1 and NP2 respectively (standing for the first and the second noun phrase). For example, in the sen-tences below the subscript identifies the preferred co-referent:

> (42) Mark *confided in* Simon because he_{Mark} had a guilty conscience.
> (43) Mark *praised* Simon because he_{Simon} had done well on the test.

In both sentences, Mark is the Agent (NP1) and Simon is the Patient (NP2). 'Confided in' therefore has NP1 preference, whereas 'praised' has NP2 preference. Essentially, the argument is that the implicit cau-sality of the main verb determines the focus of the sentence, and the focused antecedent is the one that will be the preferred co-referent of the pronoun.

Vonk (1985) found that the implicit causality of the verb had an effect on how long it took to read the subordinate clause verb phrase ('. . . had a guilty conscience') indicating that the implicit causality of the verb had an effect before the end of the sentence. She found that, when the semantic interpretation of the verb phrase agreed with the causality of the main verb, clauses were read more quickly than when there was some incongruency. So 'Mark praised Simon because he had done well on the test' was read more quickly than 'Mark praised Simon because he wanted to make friends' because the interpretation of the latter sentence goes against the implicit causality of 'praised'. A con-tinuation of a sentence with 'praised' as its main verb should concern the person being praised. 'He wanted to make friends' does not do this, and therefore this sentence will take longer to read than one which agrees with the verb's causality.

The nature of the conjunction linking the main clause to the subor-dinate clause containing the pronoun also has an effect on resolution. Ehrlich (1980) and Grober et al. (1978) found a strong shift towards NP1 assignments when the conjunction 'because' was replaced with 'but'. Compare (43) to (44) below:

> (44) Mark praised Simon but <u>he</u> was being insincere.

Here the pronoun co-refers with Mark rather than Simon. The reason-ing behind the striking effect of (44) in relation to (43) is that 'but' introduces the immediate expectation of denial into the sentence. Upon encountering 'but', we are effectively notified that what is about to follow will violate one of our assumptions, as in:

(45) Mark is very smart but he cracks up in exams.

The assumption which is being violated refers to the subject of the sentence. In (45) this is the fact that Mark, being very smart, should be good at exams. The 'but' signals that there is something about this assumption that must be denied or, as in (45), qualified. The implicit causality of the verb affects the sentential focus and hence the anaphor resolution. However, the conjunction used in the sentence can shift the implicit causality and indicate a different resolution.

SAQ 40
Think of contexts for the following verbs, and then decide whether the verbs have NP1 or NP2 preference: apologized, honoured, astonished, detested, scolded, attracted, contacted, blamed, deceived, exasperated, envied, delighted, frightened, liked, lied to, impressed, upset, scared.

Compellingness
Grober et al. (1978) also examined what happened when the 'compellingness' of the verb was altered. The assumption was that the effect of implicit causality would be altered by how mandatory the verb was perceived as being:

(46) Mark *may* telephone Ana tonight because . . .
(47) Mark *must* telephone Ana tonight because . . .

Must is more forceful than *may*. A stronger preference for NP1 assignment was found in (47) as opposed to (46). The reasoning behind this is that the strong 'must' in (47) makes the action of the verb mandatory rather than optional, and therefore the full force of the implicit causality (NP1 for the verb 'to telephone') is realized. Resolution can therefore be influenced by the action of the sentence, and how important that action is.

Any number of factors can influence the focus of a sentence, and implicit causality is simply one amongst many. Obviously, many verbs do not have any significant causality, so although this is a well researched area of sentence focus it may not be the most important. The research on discourse focus is thankfully rather more straightforward, and it is to this that we now turn.

4.3   Discourse focus

Controlling the topic of a discourse is very much what storytelling is about. Moving from one theme to the next, shifting the focus from one aspect of the story to another, is often achieved through fairly artificial means such as the chapter or numbered section. There are more elegant methods of doing this, more often the preserve of the author than the academic, and these need to be understood if we are to produce a model of how co-reference is maintained within discourse. To illustrate the complexity of changing focus, consider the extract below:

> His Majesty also carried a new rifle made for him by Joao de Lara, master of arms in the royal arsenal. The rifle is a work of art and is embellished with gold and silver. Were it to be lost, it would soon be returned to its rightful owner, for along the barrel of the rifle, in bold lettering and written in Latin, as on the pediment of the Basilica of Saint Mark's in Rome, are inscribed the words: I BELONG TO THE MONARCH. MAY GOD PROTECT DOM JOAO V. Yet some people continue to insist that rifles can speak only through the mouth of the barrel and solely in the language of gunpowder and lead. This is certainly true of ordinary rifles, such as the one used by Baltasar Mateus, alias Sete-Sois, who at this very minute is unarmed and standing quite still in the middle of the Palace Square . . .
> (Saramago, 1989)

In this short passage the author has taken us from a previously established main topic (the King of Portugal), through a linking sub-topic (first Dom Joao's rifle, then rifles in general), and finally, through the medium of this discussion about rifles, on to a new main topic (Sete-Sois, the hero of the piece). At no time are we left in any doubt as to what the focus is, even though it is constantly changing. Some progress has been made towards explaining this level of mastery, but not much.

Explicit and implicit focus

Garrod and Sanford (1990) argue that there are two levels of focus within a discourse, **explicit** and **implicit focus**. Explicit focus involves the set of people and objects actually introduced by name into the discourse. Implicit focus is a representation of the current scene in which the discourse is based, and is directly analogous to a script of an event. The scenario in implicit focus serves to offer roles which the individuals in explicit focus can map on to. Garrod and Sanford argue that individuals introduced into the discourse by name will be immediately instantiated in explicit focus, whereas those introduced by *role* (e.g. 'the waiter'), will be assigned a role in implicit focus and may only enter explicit focus indirectly. By 'slotting' such individuals into role-stereotypic positions within a script or schema, one would predict that the individual would inherit some of the prototypical properties of that role. Figure 3.2 demonstrates how explicit and implicit focus affect resolution, and Techniques Box J describes a fascinating experiment on focus and anaphoric resolution.

STORY A:
Mark was talking to the waiter in the restaurant. Ten minutes later he ...

STORY B:
Mark was talking to the waiter in the restaurant. Eight hours later he ...

Antecedents available for co-reference in the first sentence of both stories:

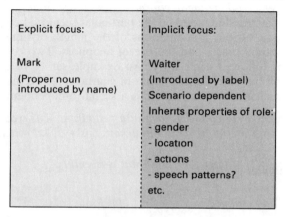

Antecedents available for co-reference after different lapses of time:

STORY A:

Explicit focus:	Implicit focus:
Mark	The waiter
(main character)	(within time frame of scenario)

STORY B:

Explicit focus:	Implicit focus:
Mark	*Empty*
(main character)	(outside time frame of scenario)

Figure 3.2   Diagram showing the operations of explicit and implicit focus. The upper box contains all the characters introduced in the first sentence of both Story A and Story B. The two lower boxes illustrate which of them are available for co-reference after different lapses of time (ten minutes in Story A or eight hours in Story B)

TECHNIQUES BOX J

Discourse Structure and Antecedent Availability
Anderson, Garrod and Sanford (1983)

Rationale
Do changes in focus (Anderson et al. refer to them as *episode shifts*) affect the availability of potential antecedents? When a main character moves out of the typical time or space in which an activity or

---

125

event occurs, are the characters in implicit focus automatically made unavailable for co-reference?

Method
Subjects were given short stories to read which contained two types of characters. One type, *main characters*, were the protagonists. The other, *scenario-dependent characters*, were peripheral participants whose existence depended on the particular scenario being acted out. There were various combinations of the length of time over which the story took place, and the use of anaphors. Two comprehension questions followed each story. An example serves to illustrate the distinction between the two types of character. Here the Browns are the main characters: the waiter is a scenario-dependent character.

The Browns were eating a meal in a restaurant. The waiter was hovering around the table. This restaurant was well known for its food.

$\left.\begin{array}{l}\textit{Five hours}\\ \textit{Forty minutes}\end{array}\right\}$ *later the restaurant was empty.*

$\left.\begin{array}{l}\textit{They}\\ \textit{He}\end{array}\right\}$ *had enjoyed* $\left\{\begin{array}{l}\textit{eating}\\ \textit{serving}\end{array}\right\}$ *the food.*

Questions:
Were the Browns eating in a restaurant?
Did the waiter enjoy serving?

Times for both reading the sentences and answering the comprehension questions were recorded. The 'time frames' of typical episodes were estimated by asking subjects who didn't take part in the main experiment to estimate the minimum and maximum time each scenario (in this case, a family eating in a restaurant) typically took. One time period ('forty minutes') was chosen to be within this time whereas the other ('five hours') was outside it. It was assumed that when subsequent action took place outside the time frame of the scenario then the scenario-dependent characters would not be available as antecedents.

Results
The results of the reading times were not all that revealing, except for an advantage for reading sentences which referred to the main as opposed to the scenario-dependent characters. However, the response times to the comprehension questions revealed an interesting pattern of results. The analysis of comprehension response times suggests that, when an episode shifts beyond its temporal or spatial 'frame', characters which were dependent on the scenario for their existence are no longer as available as when the action takes place within the frame. Therefore, co-reference is only possible when the character can be assumed to exist within the vicinity of the action, regardless of how recently he or she was mentioned.

At any point in a discourse, the preferred co-referent of an anaphor is the object or individual in focus. This is the single most important factor operating to guide anaphoric reference in discourse contexts. Focus is so important that some languages (such as Swahili) have different verb forms depending on whether the verb refers to something in focus or not. Indeed, focus may be the only factor operating at the discourse level, as all other purported influences may be reducible to focus phenomena.

SAQ 41
Go back and look at the short story we used in Section 1.2. Which of the characters are in explicit focus, and which are in implicit focus?

4.4   Anaphor antecedent distance

Because antecedents must be available in working memory, and therefore have to be actively maintained if successful and rapid resolution is to take place, it makes sense to suggest that the greater the distance between anaphor and antecedent, the harder it will be to link them together. Antecedents that are close to their anaphors are more likely to be in working memory than those which are further away. An antecedent that is far away may either have to be retrieved from the discourse representation, or may not be retrieved at all.

With regard to experiments into anaphor antecedent distance, there is again a certain amount of contradictory evidence. Whereas many studies have found that resolution time increases as a function of anaphor antecedent distance, a roughly equal number have *failed* to find an effect of distance.

What separates the two is that those studies which did not find evidence for distance effects all included a control for changes of focus. One of the problems with increasing the distance between an antecedent and an anaphor is that the intervening material can often serve to change the focus of the discourse. By changing the focus, all sorts of factors unrelated to simple distance effects may be introduced.

The question about anaphor antecedent distance may be slightly easier to answer for ellipsis. Murphy (1985) showed that antecedent distance had an effect on reading times, with ellipses that were a long way from the antecedents taking longer to read than those which were closer. Because the resolution of ellipsis requires that a memory representation of the exact wording of the antecedent clause exists, and as it is well known that memory for exact wording as opposed to gist is lost fairly quickly (Sachs, 1967), this is not surprising. This result reiterates the importance of working memory in anaphoric resolution.

As the successful resolution of ellipsis involves maintaining a verb phrase or similar chunk of information in working memory, the process may be facilitated when the antecedent is in some sense important to the discourse. This hypothesis was tested in an elegant experiment by Malt (1985), described in Techniques Box K.

TECHNIQUES BOX K

Malt (1985) and 'Important' Ellipses

Rationale

If the interpretation of ellipsis (in this experiment, verb phrase ellipsis, VPE) relies on retaining the structure of the antecedent in working memory, then indicating in some way that the antecedent will be 'important later' may be of some use in retaining the information.

Malt (1985) looked at a number of factors that might be used to aid (or hinder) the process. The most interesting of the ones she studied were question and answer pairs. If a question is left unanswered we may be left expecting an answer at a later point. A subsequent VPE which elides to the unanswered question should be easier to interpret than a VPE where the question has already been answered and is therefore no longer important.

Method

Subjects were given short stories to read off a computer screen. The subject pressed a button to advance to the next sentence, and reading times were measured by the computer. Examples of the stories are given below.

Unanswered question:
Andrea was anxious to leave the house.
'Aren't we going to the game?' she asked.
'It's getting kind of late,' she added.
'Yes, we are,' Ray assured her.

Answered question:
Andrea was anxious to leave the house.
'Aren't we going to the game?' she asked.
'It's getting kind of late,' Brian observed.
'Yes, we are,' Ray assured her.

The VPE occurred in the final sentence, 'Yes we are ø' (ø = 'going to the game'). The important difference was that in the unanswered condition Andrea had simply added another comment to her initial question. This meant that the question was left unanswered and could therefore be construed as something that might be important later and which should be held in working memory. In the answered condition, Brian's observation served as a possible answer to the question, meaning that it no longer needed to be kept active in working memory and could be discarded.

Results

The important measure was the time taken for subjects to read the final sentence, which was the one containing the ellipsis. The results are shown below.

	Unanswered condition	Answered condition
RT (millisecs)	1930	2332

As can be seen, the elliptical final sentence was read more quickly when the question containing the antecedent had not been answered, and had therefore been carried forward in memory. Another possible explanation is that, in the answered condition, the focus had shifted from Andrea to Brian, which might have made the last sentence take longer to process.

4.5   *Intonation*

One point which has emerged from all the literature reviewed to date is that a great deal of research has concerned reading as opposed to listening. As language has presumably evolved primarily in the spoken form (reading and writing are fairly recent inventions), we might expect the intonation of speech to play an important role in comprehension. Intonation often receives little more than a passing reference in textbooks on psycholinguistics, probably due to the fact that it is theoretically complex. Whilst avoiding dealing with any of these issues, we shall none the less take a brief look at how intonational context can be used to aid resolution.

The most important point about intonation is that when the focus is not evident it may serve to disambiguate a lot of the ambiguous cases we have already considered. In spoken language, the intonation and stress patterns of an utterance can serve to indicate unambiguously the correct co-referent.

Activity 2

Try saying the following sentence out loud using two different intonation patterns. The first should be what is referred to as 'default intonation'. This refers to the 'normal' reading of the sentence — fairly flat with a slight rise towards the end (. . . 'gave her the MEAsles'). The second should stress the two pronouns ('. . . SHE gave HER . . .') What happens to the pattern of resolution when you do this?

Ana gave Suzy the flu and then she gave her the measles.

Two different interpretations of this sentence exist, where the first pronoun co-refers with either Ana (in which case Ana gave Suzy the measles as well as flu), or Suzy (in which case Suzy retaliated by giving Ana measles). Contrastive stress can be used to indicate either of these two interpretations. De-emphasizing the initial 'she' indicates that Ana gave Suzy the measles, whereas emphasizing both anaphors indicates the opposite interpretation.

Bosch (1983) has put forward an interesting account of the location of antecedents which relies on ideas about stress. He argues that the way an anaphor is stressed determines where its antecedent should be located. Stressed anaphors find their antecedents in the discourse representation whereas unstressed anaphors find theirs in the linguistic representation. The sentences below illustrate this:

(48) When Mark arrived everyone ignored <u>the idiot</u>.
(49) When Mark arrived everyone ignored <u>the IDiot.</u>

Stressing 'the idiot' (a noun phrase anaphor) in (49) informs the listener that it is not Mark who is the idiot, but someone else. This someone is presumably located in the discourse representation. The normal unstressed pattern in (48) leads us to interpret 'the idiot' as co-referring with Mark.

Intonation provides useful cues which act to disambiguate spoken anaphors. In fact, many of the problems of resolution may arise because of the translation of language from auditory to written form. Perhaps the problems of anaphoric resolution are very much restricted to written language, where intonation is not available.

Summary of Section 4

- Focus is an important concept to consider when studying anaphoric co-reference. A distinction can be drawn between focus at the level of the sentence (sentential focus) and focus at the level of discourse (discourse focus).
- At the sentential level, one factor, implicit causality, has important effects on the selection of specified Agents and Patients in the first or second NP of a sentence, but these effects can be modified by the nature of the linking conjunction and the compellingness of the verb.
- At the discourse level, explicit and implicit focus refer to a distinction between explicitly named characters and implicit role characters who are only relevant in restricted scenarios.
- Other potential factors at the discourse level, like the effects of anaphor antecedent distance, can be explained as resulting from changes in focus.

• Intonation and stress may provide information which may aid in the selection of anaphors but only, of course, in spoken language.

5   The bonding process

Once the effects of linguistic sources of information, together with focus and (perhaps) intonation have been taken into account, what is there left to do? What happens at the bonding stage?

Sometimes, as it turns out, quite a lot. As most of the experimental work on anaphoric resolution has concerned antecedent activation and the effects of focus, there is little on bonding processes. However, an examination of some linguistic data does reveal that, even once an antecedent has been identified, accurate resolution is by no means guaranteed.

5.1   The final interpretation

It has been assumed throughout that the meaning of an antecedent does not change all that much when it becomes linked to an anaphor. However, identity of sense anaphors (see Section 2.4, example 30), where the meaning of an antecedent changes from a singular object to either another member of its class or the entire class of objects, demonstrates that this is not always strictly the case.

In addition, some features of ellipsis, which up until now has been described as a process of 'copying' an antecedent into the anaphoric gap, make it obvious that the relationship between the meaning of the original antecedent and that of the antecedent once linked to an anaphor is far from straightforward. To start with, it is worth stating that a literal copying process, one which merely copies the verb phrase verbatim from the antecedent position into the anaphoric gap, cannot provide a complete explanation of ellipsis. As has already been mentioned (see Section 2.3), minor changes in verb tense are tolerated. But the picture is even more complicated than this, as the form and meaning of an ellipsis can be at loggerheads with each other:

(50) Please scratch my back. Okay, then, I will ø.

SAQ 42
In the above example, what does the ellipsis refer to? Why does this prove that a literal copying process cannot work?

The story doesn't end here. Sometimes there can be quite dramatic changes to the meaning of the antecedent. The example below contains an antecedent which is copied into five elliptical gaps, changing its meaning each time:

(51) Take four eggs. Break ø into a bowl, beat ø thoroughly, season ø, fry ø for five minutes in butter, and then serve ø.

The co-referent of the four ellipses is always the same thing (the four eggs), but each anaphor refers to a different state of events. The eggs are undergoing successive changes of state between the initial and final anaphoric reference. Obviously the eggs are no longer in their shells, and have been beaten, fried, and eventually turned into an omelette.

When drawing inferences about the nature of the co-referent it is therefore necessary to take into account the *intervening context*. Even apparently small changes of wording between anaphor and antecedent can have dramatic effects on the final interpretation:

(52) It may be true of one person in one place, but not **in** <u>another</u>.
(53) It may be true of one person in one place, but not **of** <u>another</u>.

The preposition ('in' versus 'of') controls the co-reference even though the sentences are otherwise identical. This suggests that the final resolution process may involve a great deal more than simply taking an anaphor and matching it with a noun or verb phrase.

5.2   The immediacy of resolution and anaphoric ambiguity

Factors which determine whether bonding follows on immediately from selection still require careful investigation. For instance, what comes after the anaphor itself may cause us to reinterpret what we have just 'understood':

(54) Suzy asked Ana if <u>she</u> . . .
    (a) **could** leave the room.
    (b) **would** leave the room.

For most people, (54a) means that Suzy asked Ana if Suzy could leave the room (although this is ambiguous). (54b) means that Suzy asked Ana if Ana would leave the room.

As the resolution process has been split up into stages, a distinction has to be drawn between the initialization and the termination of resolution. The fact that sentences like (54a) and (54b) are unproblematic supports the idea outlined in Section 3 that, whereas selection is immediate, bonding may be delayed until more information becomes available. If the pronoun in (54) was immediately bonded with the antecedent, sentences of this type would sometimes cause garden paths. The fact that they don't suggests that it isn't.

SAQ 43
To illustrate your understanding of selection and bonding processes, take the final sentence of the last paragraph, and for the two anaphors 'they' and 'it' produce a candidate set and from this a final co-referent for each. Assuming that you understood the sentence, the final co-referents should be obvious! Also, try to identify two examples of ellipsis in the same sentence.

Of course, it may be the case that the processor is able to choose between immediacy and delay. If there are no serious contenders to the preferred antecedent, then perhaps resolution is immediate. In fact, as was suggested in Section 3.3 (p.113), if the membership of the candidate set is only one, this may itself constitute resolution. On the other hand, if there is a certain degree of doubt as to the identity of the intended co-referent, for instance if there is more than one member of the candidate set, the processor may opt to 'wait and see'. This suggests that ambiguous anaphors may be dealt with in a different way from unambiguous ones.

We have already come across a number of ambiguous anaphors. The extract below is about as good (or bad) as it gets, and offers a clear demonstration of the occasionally 'problem-solving' approach to language understanding:

> And Jacob was left alone; and there wrestled a man with him until the breaking of the day. And when he saw that he prevailed not against him, he touched the hollow of his thigh; and the hollow of Jacob's thigh was out of joint, as he wrestled with him. And he said, Let me go, for the day breaketh. And he said, I will not let thee go, except thou bless me. And he said unto him, What is thy name? And he said, Jacob.   (*Genesis*, 32: 24–7)

In order to understand this it's a good idea to start at the end, where you know who the last 'he' refers to, and work backwards. As far as I can tell, it's the angel that isn't prevailing in the second sentence.

Can we say anything sensible about how ambiguous pronouns are processed? It has already been suggested that a 'delay' strategy may come into operation, but is there anything more that can be deduced?

Let's think about what we know about pronominal resolution, and in particular the selection process. According to the multi-stage model, when a pronoun is encountered, the selection process immediately acts to select all possible antecedents of the pronoun. This list is later whittled down using downstream contextual information to end up with a single antecedent which is then bonded with the pronoun.

This general account of anaphoric resolution actually bears a striking similarity to the resolution of lexical ambiguity. Lexical ambiguity arises when an individual word in a sentence is ambiguous, and because of this the sentence has more than one meaning. Thus, in (55) the word 'bug' is ambiguous, and Mark is either putting an insect or a listening device into the room:

(55) Mark put the bug in the room.

In contrast, anaphoric ambiguity arises from an incomplete specification of the relationships that hold between anaphors and antecedents in a discourse. Anaphoric ambiguity is *stylistically* rather than linguistically problematic.

There is an analogy between the two types of ambiguity. Numerous studies of lexical ambiguity have suggested that sentence context has no effect on the selection of an ambiguous word, with context operating to select the appropriate one at a later stage (see Techniques Box E in Part II, Section 2.2). This is very similar to the way in which the co-reference processor seems to operate. The selection process selects all the possible antecedents for the anaphor, with one being subsequently bonded. If we consider 'he' below to have two distinct meanings (Mark and Simon), the analogy should become clear:

(56) Mark went shopping with Simon because <u>he</u> liked the girl who worked in Boots.

The ambiguous pronoun causes its two possible 'meanings' to be selected. One is later chosen as the co-referent, when the context makes this clear. This choice mirrors the effect of context in the resolution of lexical ambiguity.

It is interesting to see how far the analogy can be taken. Perhaps the most important difference between processing ambiguous words and ambiguous pronouns is that failure to comprehend the latter may result in serious comprehension breakdown. As a result, we might expect pronominal ambiguity to be perceived immediately. With lexical ambiguity, the perception of ambiguity is probably not a useful thing to do, especially considering the extent to which words in English have multiple meanings. A processor which was overly sensitive to lexical ambiguity would be very disruptive to rapid comprehension.

Although in the end it is not clear how far the analogy between lexical and pronominal ambiguity can be taken, the similarity between the two processes is appealing. If the initial stages of the two processes are similar, then a good starting point for an investigation of pronominal ambiguity would be an understanding of how lexical ambiguity is processed. In order to study how pronominal ambiguity is processed it is necessary to construct models of lexical ambiguity resolution. It is interesting to speculate on the possibility that ambiguous anaphors are processed in much the same way as other ambiguous words.

5.3   Anaphors and inferences

Anaphoric resolution is not an all-or-nothing process. Between encountering an anaphor and bonding it with the correct antecedent a number of things can happen. Even with an unambiguous anaphor, the inferential mechanisms required for bonding may not always occur, and this failure to process the links tying pieces of discourse together may be one of the reasons for our occasional failures to understand language.

It does seem a little strange to suggest that when the selection process produces a single candidate it is not immediately bonded with the anaphor. As further information can only really counterindicate the correct antecedent, delayed bonding seems pointless. Normal discourse does not contain vast numbers of anaphors whose antecedents are not immediately and definitely obvious. It has been pointed out on several occasions that one of the features of good discourse is co-referential clarity. The operation of a habitual delay strategy, or incomplete bonding, seems very unlikely given the weight of evidence against it. But anaphoric reference is still an inferential process, and the all-or-nothing nature of inferences in on-line comprehension is a highly contentious issue.

A distinction was drawn in Part II between *necessary* and *elaborative inferences*. Necessary inferences were defined as ones that were drawn as a consequence of the structure of the lexicon and semantic rules based on selection restrictions. Elaborative inferences were those which were dependent on context. Nothing was said about the necessity of their being drawn, although it was assumed for the most part that they were necessary for comprehension.

This distinction can be further fragmented. The notion of an elaborative inference can be split into those which are and are not *critical* in the context of the discourse. A critical inference might take the form of realizing that 'honey' in 'her hair was honey' means blond and not something made by bees.

Overall, anaphoric inferences are not mandatory. They are not completely automatic, but may involve varying degrees of search through either linguistic or discourse representations. Given that they are not in the strict sense necessary, the question arises as to whether they are *critical* or not.

Selectional inferences (the workings of the selection process) would seem to be automatic and immediate, and therefore necessary. However, the final bonding process may not be necessary. Oakhill, Garnham and Vonk (1989) argue that resolution of a name with a pronoun is only achieved if demanded by the context (for instance, when you are asked a question that concerns resolution), and that otherwise bonding does not occur. They suggest that co-reference is not as important as **cohesion**. Cohesion involves role mapping (figuring out what did what) and they argue that this is more important than name mapping (understanding who did what). Take (57) as an example:

(57) Mark praised Simon because <u>he</u> had done well on the test.

The co-reference process would bond 'he' with 'Simon' (Section 4.2 examines why this potentially ambiguous anaphor is interpreted so easily). The cohesion process, on the other hand, simply needs to note that one person is being praised, and that this is because that same person had done well on a test. The actual names of the people involved are not important. Of course, co-reference and cohesion often go hand in hand, but Oakhill et al. argue that they aren't necessarily dependent on one another.

Role to role mapping (cohesion) would therefore seem to fall into the category of elaborative inferences which *have* to be drawn. Role to name mapping inferences (anaphor resolution) are not so important. Therefore the bonding inference is *not* critical for comprehension, and full anaphoric reference may not always take place.

Summary of Section 5

- Anaphoric resolution is not as simple as extracting an antecedent from a discourse and linking it with an anaphor. The meaning of an antecedent may change as a result of information occurring either before or after the anaphor.
- Anaphoric ambiguity is similar to lexical ambiguity. Although the processes involved may be very different, the patterns of lexical and pronominal ambiguity resolution seem to mirror one another.
- Although linking concepts across and within sentences is crucial for understanding language, it is possible that *cohesion* is more important than co-reference, and therefore that the full resolution of anaphor with name, as opposed to anaphor with role, may not always occur. Many anaphors may be left only partially resolved in normal comprehension.

6   *Conclusions*

Anaphoric reference is the glue that holds language understanding together. It links what is being said at the moment to that which has already passed. The use of anaphors is essentially one that appeals to simplicity — replace ideas, persons or concepts with simple labels so that when they need to be referred to in future this can be achieved with a simple phrase or even a single word rather than a reiteration of all the facts, figures and details which adhere to them. Considering the performance limitations of the human sentence processing mechanism, principally those of working memory, anaphors prevent language from becoming hopelessly unwieldy.

It has been pointed out on several occasions that, although the *description* of anaphoric reference is perfectly straightforward, the *process* by which anaphor and antecedent are linked is not. Anaphoric reference is not always as simple as pulling a label out of the discourse and linking it to a pronoun. Antecedents do not always reside in the linguistic context, and in order to produce a comprehensive theory of language understanding we need to take account of more than just the words that have been spoken. Language understanding is about the active construction of models, and it is only by understanding how these models are constructed, and what they 'look like' that we can understand how anaphoric reference, and the rest of language understanding, is achieved.

SAQ 44
There is an ellipsis in the first sentence of the final paragraph ('It has been pointed out ...'). Try to identify where it occurs, and what the antecedent is.

In conclusion, we need to ask what it means to comprehend a discourse or sentence. There is a definite intuitive feeling about understanding, but it is hard to relate this to any one *level* of understanding. We can read a page of a book and be aware of understanding the meaning of all the words, and perhaps of each individual sentence, but still not have a clue about what the page was about. Furthermore, a novel may be *allegorical*; you may read it and understand the story at face value, but when the allegory is explained you immediately understand it at another, deeper level. Does this mean you didn't understand it the first time round? Obviously not, as the perception and feeling of comprehension were there all the time. None the less, it is still reasonable to suggest that you didn't really understand the *full* meaning of the book.

Comprehension may have as much to do with phenomenology (conscious experience) as language. It is not enough just to say a sentence or a piece of text has been comprehended. We need a deeper understanding of what is meant by comprehension. Normally, the term has been used in an all-or-nothing way. You either understand something or you don't. In Part I, Section 5.4, it was claimed that we need to make inferences in order to understand language. Not everything is handed to us on a plate (even a spinning one), and it is not enough just to know how language users draw inferences. We must also examine how we know *which* inferences to draw.

Returning to one of the points made at the start of this part, anaphoric resolution seems immediate and effortless. As the numerous experiments and examples contained in this part demonstrate, this does not mean that nothing interesting happens between encountering an anaphor and deciding what it co-refers with. There are some linguistic rules which seem to guide this process, but they are not always adhered to and in any case are not sufficient for understanding to take place. Even when an antecedent has been selected, the task of resolution is not as simple as bonding it with the anaphor. The relationship between the meaning of something when it is first introduced and when it is used anaphorically is extremely complex, and remains one of the most absorbing challenges for a complete theory of anaphoric resolution.

Overview

Judith Greene

Because language is such a pervasive element in human behaviour, it is exceedingly difficult to divide it up into separate topics. So, as you have probably realized, the three parts of this book go over a lot of the same ground. Part I draws attention to the role of different types of knowledge in language understanding. Parts II and III consider how different types of knowledge are involved in language processing.

It is equally difficult to separate language from other cognitive processes involved in thinking, remembering and acting. You may, indeed, have been wondering why a book on language understanding seems to concentrate as much on knowledge and rules stored in memory as on language understanding itself. This is because cognitive psychologists are interested in the question of how the competence to use a language is represented in memory. Their concern is with language use in its widest communicative sense, often blurring the traditional distinction between linguistic competence and linguistic performance.

This Overview will present a cross-section of some of the main themes raised throughout the book in order to bring together aspects of language that were originally introduced in different sections.

1 Types of knowledge

A brief list of the knowledge available to language users would include at least the following:

1 The lexicon (i.e. rules for mapping sounds and written letters on to representations of word meanings). The question of whether these should be represented as lists of semantic features, case frames or semantic primitives was discussed in Part I, Section 2.
2 Syntactic rules (i.e. grammatical rules which specify how words should be combined). See Part I, Section 3 for a description of Chomsky's transformational grammar, and Part II, Section 3 for the implementation of syntactic parsers, such as Augmented Transition Networks (ATNs).
3 Semantic rules (i.e. rules for combining individual word meanings into sentence interpretations). Part II, Section 2 is concerned with the problem of selecting appropriate word senses in a sentence context.
4 General knowledge about the world (i.e. knowledge about objects and events, procedures and experiences). This type of script-based

knowledge is assumed to underlie the understanding of discourse, and of the topics in focus (See Part I, Section 5; Part II, Section 4; and Part III, Section 4.)

2 Language processing

As indicated in the Introduction, one major theme is the extent to which language processing involves separate processing modules which are independent of each other.

Independent models

The linear model described in Part II, Section 1.2 assumes that there are independent processing stages in language understanding. In Figure 2.1 there are separate modules for lexical processing, syntactic processing and semantic processing. In Part III, Section 3, there is a similar multi-stage model shown in Figure 3.1, but here the main distinction is between linguistic processes and a stage where non-linguistic processes invoking general knowledge are operating.

One major method for testing independence is by means of cross-modal priming experiments. If there is access to word senses regardless of context, this implies that there is independent access during the linguistic processing of a sentence. The argument is that it is only after processing of a sentence is completed that information derived from other types of processing comes into play.

Interactive models

The interactive model described in Part II, Section 1.3 takes the opposite view that, since humans have access to all kinds of knowledge, they will exploit whatever information is most helpful when selecting a plausible meaning for a sentence. The model in Figure 2.2 in Part II is equivalent to the single stage model in Figure 3.1 in Part III. In both cases, it is assumed that all types of information are available when selecting a sentence meaning based on appropriate links between words, including anaphors.

The claim is made in Part II that many of the attempts to write language understanding computer programs have found it necessary to allow the program to consult other sources of information in an interactive mode, as in Cottrell's model and Winograd's model. St John's model is explicitly based on the non-linguistic knowledge embodied in scripts. Similarly, Part III, Sections 3.4 and 3.5 give examples of when the selection of anaphoric antecedents appears to draw on discourse knowledge, while Section 4 describes experiments in which knowledge about the topic of a discourse and the allocation of script-based roles can affect the interpretation of anaphors in the bonding process.

The effects of different types of information at various stages of language processing are still problematical. The time-course of sentence processing is dependent on the milliseconds required to access and select combinations of word meanings. Language processing appears to be so instantaneous for fluent speakers and readers that it is difficult to pinpoint particular stages. Nevertheless, new experimental techniques and more sophisticated computer programs have thrown light on the intricacies of language processing.

3 Language as a psychological activity

So where does all this leave psychological theories of language? It seems obvious enough that linguistic knowledge must be stored in long-term memory and that linguistic processing goes on in some kind of short-term working memory. But do we, as Noam Chomsky suggests, have a separate linguistic competence? Or is our ability to use language part of our general ability to respond to the world about us? Language does not occur in a vacuum but involves all our cognitive abilities and stored knowledge about the world.

As you might expect, human language users are normally more interested in the situations being described than in linguistic intricacies. When we are conversing in a language we know well, we seem to be speaking our thoughts directly, presenting the content of arguments rather than making linguistic decisions. The words on a page seem to 'speak' to us directly: the purpose of talking is to say what we mean. Yet this natural 'transparency' of language can be all too easily shattered when we attempt to express complex thoughts on paper. In these circumstances, words and phrases seem to take on an obstinate life of their own.

The same is true when we try to learn another language. Despite all the general knowledge that speakers may have in common, communication is very limited without a shared language. Acquiring a new language involves learning a whole new linguistic system, including vocabulary, grammar, idioms and conversational conventions. As with other highly learned skills, once truly mastered, the linguistic apparatus seems to disappear, allowing us to concentrate on the interpretation of meanings and intentions. As they acquire competence, speakers move from the level of word meanings, through sentence meanings, to interpretations of discourses, until they can use a language to communicate everything they want to express. It is at this stage, when language and meanings have become inextricably mixed, that it becomes impossible to distinguish the relative roles of language and thought. Do the particular languages we speak constrain the way we think or is language a neutral tool for expressing our thoughts?

There are many concepts which seem to be universal to all human beings (e.g. semantic 'primitives' like 'cause', 'transfer of possession', 'move', 'ingest', and so on). Whatever the special customs of a society, its members are likely to want to talk about eating, giving and moving around. But a restaurant script may be particular to eating customs in American restaurants rather than to eating habits in all human societies. So language seems to depend both on universal knowledge shared by all human beings and on highly specific knowledge restricted to a particular society. All we can be sure of is that language simultaneously reflects and shapes our attitudes and actions within the society in which we live.

The exact relationship between linguistic skills, general knowledge and communication is mysterious indeed. Psychological investigations and computer models continue to reveal the incredible cognitive abilities and knowledge taken for granted by every language user. It is this multi-faceted nature of human language that guarantees it a central position in cognitive psychology.

Answers to SAQs

SAQ 1
(a) *Visiting aunts can be a nuisance* can either mean (i) that having to go and visit aunts can be a nuisance or (ii) that aunts who visit can be a nuisance.
(b) The girls would assume meaning (ii); that is, that aunts must be visiting them.
(c) Meaning (i) because the aunts cannot go out to visit anyone.

SAQ 2
(a) Possible sentences would be *The violinist displayed a masterly use of his bow* and *At the end of the concert the violinist took a bow.*
(b) *Bank* can mean the edge of a river, a place for money transactions, an aeroplane turning.

SAQ 3
Possible synonym phrases might be:
(a) *made a present of*
(b) *phoned*
(c) *infected . . . with*
(d) *surrendered*
(e) *resigned.*

SAQ 4
Bachelor (+ human)(+ adult)(– married). One problem with semantic features is how to explain combinations like *bachelor girl, bachelor apartment,* or why it sounds rather odd to say *The Pope is a well-known bachelor*, although he is an unmarried adult male.

SAQ 5
(a) Agent: *John*   Object: *window*   Instrument: *hammer*
(b) Instrument: *hammer*   Object: *window*
(c) Agent: *John*   Recipient: *Mary*   Location: *party.*
Note that there is an implied, but non-stated, Agent in (b), i.e. the person who used or threw the hammer to break the window, and a non-stated Object in (c), probably either an invitation card or a verbal invitation.

SAQ 6
(a) ATRANS
(b) MTRANS
(c) PTRANS
(d) INGEST
(e) MOVE
(f) MBUILD

Answers to SAQs

SAQ 7

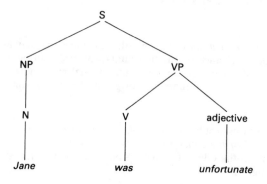

SAQ 8

Sentences (a) and (b) have the same deep structures representing the identical meaning that a new student painted the picture. Sentences (b) and (c) have similar surface structures (i.e. the order of the words is much the same) but quite different deep structures. Sentence (c) has the different meaning that someone painted a picture using a new technique.

SAQ 9

Sentence (a) should be the easiest because it is 'irreversible' according to our usual expectations of doctor/patient relationships. Sentence (b) is considered to be 're-versible', although in our society there may be a slight expectation that a boy is more likely to kiss a girl than the other way round! Sentence (c) should take the longest because it contradicts our expectations. In fact, quite a few of Herriot's subjects misread it to mean that the lifeguard saved the bather, indicating that they were influenced by semantic expectations rather than carrying out a prior syntactic analysis.

SAQ 10

Semantic features; semantic cases; semantic primitives.

SAQ 11

(a) The subject of *admire* has to have the feature (+ human) so as to allow *John admires the picture* but to rule out *The picture admires John*.
(b) There are so many possible objects of *admire*, (e.g. *I admire John, I admire jazz, I admire courage*) that it is difficult to know what selection restrictions are needed. Perhaps *admire* just needs the features: subject (+ human) and object (+ admirable).

SAQ 12

(a) Acceptable as meaning 'strike' because Peter is (+ human) and the object (rock) and instrument (ball) are both (+ physical object).
(b) Not acceptable, because the sense of hit meaning 'strike' requires (+ human) subject.
(c) Acceptable for 'collide', because Peter is (+ human) (+ physical object) and so the rock (+ physical object) can 'collide' with him.

(d) Acceptable for both meanings of *hit*, because John is (+ human) for 'strike' but both John and Peter are (+ physical object) and so could 'collide'. However, I think you would agree that most people would assume the 'strike' sense, especially in the context of a dance!

SAQ 13
Some actions which most of Bower et al.'s subjects agreed about include: wake up, get up, dress, eat breakfast, brush teeth, leave house.

SAQ 14
(a) The bridging inference is that beer was being taken to be drunk at the picnic.
(b) It is general knowledge that drinks like beer are drunk at picnics, that picnics are generally held on hot days in the summer and so beer kept in the boot of a car is likely to get warm.

SAQ 15
The listener at the end of the telephone can still hear the intonation and emphasis of the speaker's voice. But the speaker and the listener cannot see each other's facial expressions and gestures and they are not present in the same situation. The message may also be acoustically distorted.

SAQ 16
(a) A priming context for *butter* would be the word *bread*.
(b) A neutral context word would be *doctor*.

SAQ 17
The response in (a) should be faster than that in (b) because the word *nurse* is associated with the word *doctor*. The word *postman* should not have any priming effect on the word *doctor*.

SAQ 18
(a) A possible context sentence for priming the meaning of *spade* which would facilitate the target word *tool* would be: *You should have worked with a spade.*
(b) A possible control sentence would be: *You should have worked in the shop.* Only (a) would be expected to prime the target word *tool*.

SAQ 19

Game	Agents	Instruments
SNOOKER	Two players and a referee	Cues and coloured balls
BRIDGE	Four players	Pack of cards
SOCCER	22 players, referee and two linesmen	Ball

SAQ 20

PAGT	Agents who can propel	*Bob or John*
PROPEL	Act of propelling	*threw*
POBJ	Objects which can be propelled	*a ball*
PREC	Agents who can be recipients of propelled objects	*John or Bob*

145

Answers to SAQs

SAQ 21
(a) There is nothing wrong with the syntax.
(b) The dog which is being chased by the cat is described as 'black' (*the black dog*) and also as 'brown' (*is brown*), which is semantically unacceptable.
(c) It is not very likely that a cat would be chasing a dog rather than the other way round.

SAQ 22
(a) *I bought a watch.* (target word: CLOCK)
(b) *They decided to watch.* (target word: CLOCK)

SAQ 23
(a) A correct analysis by the parser would be that it is the dog which is being chased by the bull.
(b) Syntactic cues would include the *active form* of the first verb which indicates that the dog is chasing the cat and the *passive form* of the second verb which indicates that someone is being chased by a bull. The use of the word *which* indicates that *which is chasing the cat* is a subordinate clause and so identifies *the dog* as being the subject of *is being chased by the bull.*

SAQ 24
(a) Rule 1 (article *the* and noun *boy*).
(b) Adjective loop (adjective *big*, adjective *blue* and noun *blocks*).
(c) Rule 4 (pronoun *she*).
(d) Rule 1 and adjective loop (article *the*, adjective *tall*, adjective *bright*, and noun *child*).

SAQ 25
Strategies (1) to (3) are within the syntactic component because they are concerned with how the parser operates. Strategies (4) and (5) involve interacting with other components, semantics and general knowledge.

SAQ 26
Likely garden path interpretation:
(a) An unknown assassin.
(b) The prince.
(c) The death of the prince.
Interpretation of whole sentence:
(a) The prince.
(b) Probably birds.
(c) The bad shooting performance of the prince.

SAQ 27
(a) *John went down the road (in a bus).*
(b) *John went down (the road in a bus).*
Of course, humans would not even consider option (b) which implies that John was walking down a road which was in a bus. However, language understanding computer programs have to be given precise instructions about how to parse sentences like these.

SAQ 28
There are many such inferences in the paraphrase, including the fact that John sat down, read the menu, ate the lobster, paid the bill and left the restaurant. All these are inferences about events which are not mentioned in the story. The paraphrase is, of course, extremely boring, but the purpose of these inferences is to enable SAM to answer questions like *Who gave John the lobster?*

SAQ 29

Clement	paid	the bill
Agent	Action	Patient

SAQ 30
1 One of the sentences in the text states that the restaurant was expensive.
2 It is stated that Clement paid the bill, so it is inferred that he did the tipping.
3 Based on prior experience of Clement, the program identifies him as (.6) likely to order cheap wine and therefore he can be inferred to be mean (or poor!).

On the basis of these inferences the program decides that, because Clement paid the bill (.9), he would also be tipping (.9), and obviously he would be tipping the waiter (.9). Although the restaurant is expensive, it is known that Clement is mean. Therefore, as a result of these two conflicting bits of information, the probability of Clement giving a small tip is (.4).

SAQ 31
The story is reproduced below, with all the anaphors underlined. If you did not spot all of them, don't worry. There are a number of different types of anaphor, the main kinds of which are examined in Section 2.

> Ana was going on holiday with Mark and Simon. <u>She</u> was going to lie on the beach doing nothing for two weeks. <u>Mark</u> had been in charge of all the arrangements, <u>he</u> had booked them a flight that left at four in the afternoon. When <u>they</u> got to the airport a stewardess told <u>them</u> that fog was delaying the departure of <u>their</u> plane. After a long wait <u>they</u> finally boarded <u>the plane</u>. <u>Ana</u> was first up the steps where the pilot was waiting to meet <u>them</u>.
> 'Hello', <u>she</u> said, 'I hope <u>we</u> manage to take off in all <u>this fog</u>.'
> 'I'm sure there'll be no problem', came the reply.

SAQ 32
(a) The anaphor is 'he', the co-referent is 'the burglar.'
(b) The anaphor is 'she', the co-referent is 'Suzy.'
(c) The anaphors are 'she' and 'it', and their respective co-referents are 'Ana' and 'the dog.'

SAQ 33
Sentence (12) could be preceded with something like 'Ana had been shopping the previous day'. Sentence (13) makes sense if you precede it with something along the lines of 'A woman and her friend had both put their things into one handbag'.

SAQ 34
The ellipsis occurs at the end of the second sentence. 'Yes I am ø.' (ø = 'going to the concert.')

Answers to SAQs

SAQ 35
'...which they are ø.' (ø = 'less than total') A syntactic reading of this suggests that his loyalty is less than total. Presumably the intended meaning was the opposite of this.

SAQ 36
It is ø. Are you ø? In both cases, ø = 'independent'.

SAQ 37
The deictic interpretation refers to the case where Ana and Suzy are talking about someone else who is not mentioned in the text, and how they like her hair. In this case, the someone else's hair is the deictic co-referent of both 'her hair' and 'it'.

SAQ 38
'She' is also commonly used to refer to things like cars and ships. In addition to 'singular, female', we might like to say that 'she' can co-refer with objects that have the features 'large, mechanical' as well.

SAQ 39
The phenomenon is called *false bonding*. See the end of Section 3.3.

SAQ 40
Agreement is usually fairly high about these, but don't worry if you disagree about a couple of them. Normally, *apologized, astonished, attracted, contacted, deceived, exasperated, delighted, frightened, lied to, impressed, upset,* and *scared* are interpreted as NP1 verbs, whereas *honoured, detested, liked, scolded, envied,* and *blamed* are NP2.

SAQ 41
Explicit focus contains all the antecedents introduced by *name* (i.e. Ana, Mark and Simon). Implicit focus contains those introduced by *role* (in this case, the pilot and the stewardess).

SAQ 42
The ellipsis refers to 'my back', except that 'my back' is not *my* back, but the back of the person who wants their back scratched. A tricky point, but an important one. If you interpreted this using a pure copying process you would probably be accused of being facetious.

SAQ 43
With 'they', the candidate set would consist of 'sentences' and 'garden paths', with 'sentences' being finally chosen. For 'it' the process would select 'pronoun' and 'antecedent', with 'pronoun' being the final choice. There are two ellipses in the sentence: '...they don't ø' (ø = 'cause garden paths'); and '...it isn't ø' (ø = 'bonded with the antecedent').

SAQ 44
The ellipsis occurs at the end of the sentence: '...are linked is not ø' (ø = 'perfectly straightforward').

References

ANDERSON, A., GARROD, S.C. and SANFORD, A.J. (1983) 'The accessibility of pronominal antecedents as a function of episode shifts in narrative text', *Quarterly Journal of Experimental Psychology*, 35A, pp.427–40.

BLACK, J.B. and WILENSKY, R. (1979) 'An evaluation of story grammars', *Cognitive Science*, 3, pp.213–29.

BOWER, G.H., BLACK J.B. and TURNER, T.J. (1979) 'Scripts in text comprehension and memory', *Cognitive Psychology*, 11, pp.177–220.

BOSCH, P. (1983) *Agreement and Anaphora: A Study of the Role of Pronouns in Syntax and Discourse*, Academic Press.

BRANSFORD, J.D. and JOHNSON, M.K. (1972) 'Contextual prerequisites for understanding: some investigations of comprehension and recall', *Journal of Verbal Learning and Verbal Behavior*, 11, pp.717–26.

BROADBENT, D.E. (1973) *In Defence of Empirical Psychology*, Methuen.

BROWN, G. and YULE, G. (1983) *Discourse Analysis*, Cambridge University Press.

CLARK, H.H. (1977) 'Bridging', in JOHNSON-LAIRD, P.N. and WASON, P.C. (eds) *Thinking: Readings in Cognitive Science*, Cambridge University Press.

CLARK, H.H. and MURPHY, G.L. (1982) 'Audience design in meaning and reference', in LE NY, J.F. and KINTSCH, W. (eds) *Language and Comprehension*, North Holland.

CHOMSKY, N. (1957) *Syntactic Structures*, Mouton.

CHOMSKY, N. (1965) *Aspects of the Theory of Syntax*, MIT press.

COHEN, G. (1983) *The Psychology of Cognition* (2nd edn), Academic Press.

COTTRELL, G.W. (1989) *A Connectionist Approach to Word Sense Disambiguation*, Pitman.

COULSON, M.C. (1991) *The Use and Processing of Pronominal Anaphora in English*, unpublished Ph.D. thesis, Cambridge University.

CRAIN, S. and STEEDMAN, M.J. (1985) 'On not being led up the garden path: the use of context by the psychological parser', in DOWTY, D., KARTTUNEN, L. and ZURICKY, A. (eds) *Natural Language Parsing*, Cambridge University Press.

CRAWLEY, R.A. and STEVENSON, R.J. (1990) 'Reference in single sentences and in texts', *Journal of Psycholinguistic Research*, 19, pp.191–210.

EHRLICH, K. (1980) 'Comprehension of pronouns', *Quarterly Journal of Experimental Psychology*, 32, pp.247–55.

FILLMORE, C.J. (1968) 'The case for case', in BACH, E. and HARMS, R.T. (eds) *Universals in Linguistic Theory*, Holt, Rinehart and Winston.

FLETCHER, C.R. (1984) 'Markedness and topic continuity in discourse processing', *Journal of Verbal Learning and Verbal Behavior*, 23, pp.487–93.

FOSS, D.J. and HAWKES, D.T. (1978) *Psycholinguistics*, Holt, Rinehart and Winston.

GARNHAM, A. (1985) *Psycholinguistics: Central Topics*, Methuen.

GARNHAM, A. and OAKHILL, J. (1987) 'Interpreting elliptical verb phrases', *Quarterly Journal of Experimental Psychology*, 39A, pp.611–28.

References

GARNHAM, A. and OAKHILL, J. (1989) 'The everyday use of anaphoric expressions: implications for the "mental models" theory of text comprehension', in SHARKEY, N.E. (ed.) *Models of Cognition: An Annual Review of Cognitive Science*, Volume 1, Ablex.

GARROD, S. and SANFORD, A.J. (1990) 'Referential processing in reading: focussing on roles and individuals', in BALOTA, D.A., FLORES D'ARCAIS, G.B. and RAYNER, K. (eds) *Comprehension Processes in Reading*, Lawrence Erlbaum Associates.

GERNSBACHER, M.A. (1990) 'Comprehending conceptual anaphors', *Language and Cognitive Processes*, 6, pp.81–106.

GREENE, J. (1972) *Psycholinguistics: Chomsky and Psychology*, Penguin Books.

GREENE, J. (1975) *Thinking and Language*, Methuen.

GREENE, J. (1986) *Language Understanding: A Cognitive Approach*, Open University Press in association with The Open University (Open Guides to Psychology Series).

GRINDER, J.T. and POSTAL, P.M. (1971) 'Missing antecedents', *Linguistic Inquiry*, 2, pp.269–312.

GRISHMAN, R. (1986) *Computational Linguistics: An Introduction*, Cambridge University Press.

GROBER, E.H., BEARDSLEY, W. and CARAMAZZA, A. (1978) 'Parallel function strategy in pronoun assignment', *Cognition*, 6, pp.117–33.

HERRIOT, P. (1969) 'The comprehension of active and passive sentences as a function of pragmatic expectations', *Journal of Verbal Learning and Verbal Behavior*, 8, pp.166–9.

HIRST, G. (1981) *Anaphora in Natural Language and Understanding: A Survey*, Springer-Verlag.

KAHNEY, H. (1993) *Problem Solving: Current Issues*, Open University Press in association with The Open University (Open Guides to Psychology series).

KATZ, J.J. and FODOR, J.A. (1963) 'The structure of a semantic theory', *Language*, 39, pp.170–210.

LYONS, J. (1981) *Language, Meaning and Context*, Penguin Books.

MALT, B.C. (1985) 'The role of discourse structure in understanding anaphora', *Journal of Memory and Language*, 24, pp.271–89.

MANDLER, J.M. and JOHNSON, N.S. (1977) 'Rememberance of things parsed: story structure and recall', *Cognitive Psychology*, 9, pp.111–51.

MARCUS, M.P. (1980) *A Theory of Syntactic Recognition for Natural Language*, MIT Press.

MARSLEN-WILSON, W.D., LEVY, E. and TYLER, W.K. (1981) 'Producing interpretable discourse: the establishment and maintenance of reference', in JARVELLA, R.J. and KLEIN, W. (eds) *Speech, Place and Action*, John Wiley.

MEYER, D.E. and SCHVANEVELDT, R.W. (1971) 'Facilitation in recognizing pairs of words: evidence of a dependence between retrieval operations', *Journal of Experimental Psychology*, 90, pp.227–34.

MILNE, R. (1982) 'Predicting garden path sentences', *Cognitive Science*, 6, pp.349–73.

MURPHY, G.L. (1985) 'Processes of understanding anaphora', *Journal of Memory and Language*, 24, pp.290–303.

NICOL, J. (1988) *Co-reference Processing During Sentence Comprehension*, unpublished Ph.D. dissertation, MIT.

OAKHILL, J., GARNHAM, A. and VONK, W. (1989) 'The on-line construction of discourse models', *Language and Cognitive Processes*, 4, pp.263–86.

PARSONS, D. (1969) *Funny Amusing and Funny Amazing*, Pan Books.

PINKER, S. (1994) *The Language Instinct*, Penguin Books.

POSTAL, P.M. (1969) 'Anaphoric islands', *Chicago Linguistics Society*, 5, pp.205–39.

RITCHIE, G. and THOMPSON, H. (1984) in O'SHEA, T. and EISENSTADT, M. *Artificial Intelligence: Tools, Techniques and Applications*, Harper and Row.

SACHS, J. (1967) 'Recognition memory for syntactic and semantic aspects of connected discourse', *Perception and Psychophysics*, 2, pp.437–42.

SANFORD, A.J. and GARROD, S.C. (1989) 'What, when, and how?: questions of immediacy in anaphoric reference resolution', *Language and Cognitive Processes*, 4, pp.235–62.

SARAMAGO, J. (1989) *Baltasar and Blimunda*, Picador.

SCHANK, R.C. (1972) 'Conceptual dependency: a theory of natural language understanding', *Cognitive Psychology*, 3, pp.552–631.

SCHANK, R.C. (1982) *Reading and Understanding: Teaching from the Perspective of Artificial Intelligence*, Lawrence Erlbaum.

SCHANK, R.C. and ABELSON, R.P. (1977) *Scripts, Plans, Goals and Understanding*, Lawrence Erlbaum.

SEARLE, J. (1970) *Speech Acts*, Cambridge University Press.

SEIDENBERG, M.S., TANENHAUS, M., LEIMAN, J. and BIENKOWSKI, M. (1982) 'Automatic access of the meanings of ambiguous words in context: some limitations of knowledge-based processing', *Cognitive Psychology*, 14, pp.489–537.

SLOBIN, D. (1966) 'Grammatical transformations and sentence comprehension in childhood and adulthood', *Journal of Verbal Learning and Verbal Behavior*, 5, pp.219–27.

ST JOHN, M.F. (1992) 'The story gestalt: a model of knowledge-intensive processes in text comprehension', *Cognitive Science*, 16, pp.271–306.

STEVENSON, R.J. and VITKOVITCH, M. (1986) 'The comprehension of anaphoric relations', *Language and Speech*, 29, pp.335–60.

TYLER, L.K. and MARSLEN-WILSON, W.D. (1983) 'Processing utterances in discourse contexts: on-line resolution of anaphors', *Journal of Semantics*, 1, pp.297–314.

VAN DIJK, T.A. and KINTSCH, W. (1983) *Strategies of Discourse Comprehension*, Academic Press.

VILLAUME, W.A. (1988) 'Interaction, involvement and the use of referential and formal anaphora in conversation', *Language and Speech*, 31, pp.357–74.

VONK, W. (1985) 'On the purpose of reading and the immediacy of processing pronouns', in GRONER, R., McCONKIE, G.W. and MENZ, C. (eds) *Eye Movements and Human Information Processing*, North Holland.

WINOGRAD, T. (1972) *Understanding Natural Language*, Academic Press.

WINOGRAD, T. (1980) 'What does it mean to understand language?', *Cognitive Science*, 4, pp.209–41.

References

WINOGRAD, T. and FLORES, F. (1986) *Understanding Computers and Cognition*, Ablex.

WOODS, W.A. (1970) 'Transition network grammars for natural language analysis', *Communications of the Association for Computing Machinery*, 13, p.591.

Index of Authors

Anderson, A., Garrod, S.C. and
  Sanford, A.J. (1983)   125–6

Black, J.B. and Wilkensky, R.
  (1979)   41
Bower, G.H., Black, J.B. and Turner,
  T.J. (1979)   42–3
Bosch, P. (1983)   130
Bransford, J.D. and Johnson, M.K.
  (1972)   45–7
Broadbent, D.E. (1973)   119
Brown, G. and Yule, G. (1983)   121

Clark, H.H. (1977)   45
Clark, H.H. and Murphy, G.L. (1982)
  77
Chomsky, N. (1957)   28–30, 33
Chomsky, N. (1965)   18, 31–2
Cohen, G. (1983)   49
Cottrell, G.W. (1989)   67–9, 89
Coulson, M.C. (1991)   114
Crain, S. and Steedman, M.J. (1985)
  77
Crawley, R.A. and Stevenson, R.J.
  (1990)   121

Ehrlich, K. (1980)   122

Fillmore, C.J. (1968)   25–6
Fletcher, C.R. (1984)   120
Foss, D.J. and Hawkes, D.T. (1978)
  76

Garnham, A. (1985)   49, 70, 89
Garnham, A. and Oakhill, J. (1987)
  117
Garnham, A. and Oakhill, J. (1989)
  102
Garrod, S. and Sanford, A.J. (1990)
  124
Gernsbacher, M.A. (1990)   116
Greene, J. (1972)   49
Greene, J. (1975)   49
Greene, J. (1986)   57, 89
Grinder, J.T. and Postal, P.M. (1971)
  104
Grishman, R. (1986)   116
Grober, E.H., Beardsley, W. and
  Caramazza, A. (1978)   122–3

Herriot, P. (1969)   81
Hirst, G. (1981)   120

Kahney, H. (1993)   93
Katz, J.J. and Fodor, J.A. (1963)   25

Lyons, J. (1981)   103

Malt, B.C. (1985)   128–9
Mandler, J.M. and Johnson, N.S.
  (1977)   41
Marcus, M.P. (1980)   76
Marslen-Wilson, W.D., Levy, E. and
  Tyler, W.K. (1981)   120
Meyer, D.E. and Schvaneveldt, R.W.
  (1971)   59–61
Milne, R. (1982)   76
Murphy, G.L. (1985)   127

Nicol, J. (1988)   111–12

Oakhill, J., Garnham, A. and Vonk,
  W. (1989)   135–6

Parsons, D. (1969)   77
Pinker, S. (1994)   89
Postal, P.M. (1969)   114–15

Ritchie, G. and Thompson, H. (1984)
  39

Sachs, J. (1967)   127
Sanford, A.J. and Garrod, S.C. (1989)
  113
Saramago, J. (1989)   124
Schank, R.C. (1972)   26–7
Schank, R.C. (1982)   24, 49
Schank, R.C. and Abelson, R.P.
  (1977)   42, 82–3, 85–6, 88, 97
Searle, J. (1970)   21
Seidenberg, M.S., Tanenhaus, M.,
  Leiman, J. and Bienkowski, M.
  (1982)   63–4, 71–2
Slobin, D. (1966)   33, 70
St John, M.F. (1992)   83–7, 88
Stevenson, R.J. and Vitkovitch, M.
  (1986)   108–9, 110

Tyler, L.K. and Marslen-Wilson, W.D.
  (1983)   109–10

Index of Authors

Van Dijk, T.A. and Kintsch, W.
  (1983)   42, 44
Villaume, W.A. (1988)   102–3
Vonk, W. (1985)   122

Winograd, T. (1972)   78–80
Winograd, T. (1980)   80
Winograd, T. and Flores, F. (1986)   80
Woods, W.A. (1970)   73–4

Index of Concepts

Acts 26
Anaphoric islands 114–15
Anaphoric reference 93
Anaphors 93
Antecedent 97
Audience design 77
Augmented transition networks
  (ATNs) 76

Bonding 113
Bottom-up processing 55
Bridging inferences 45

Case frames 37
Case grammar 25–6
Case slots 37
Coherence inferences 83
Cohesion 135
Competence 18
Computer models 57
Co-refer 97
Co-reference processor 97
Co-referent 97
Corpus 84
Cross-modal priming 61

Deictic anaphor 103
Deictic context 103
Deep structure 31
Deixis 103
Delayed processing 57
Discourse 40
Discourse analysis 21
Discourse focus 121
Discourse model 114

Elaborative inferences 47, 81
Ellipsis 101
Epicene pronouns 116
Explicit focus 124
Exploded cases 67

False bonding 113
Focus 95–6

Garden path sentences 76
Global focus 120

Heterarchical model 80

Identity of reference 104
Identity of sense 104
Implicit causality 122
Implicit focus 124
Inflections 19
Information processing framework
  54
Interactive model 56

Language processor 53
Lexical decision task 59
Lexical item 23
Lexical meanings 19
Lexicon 19, 23
Linear model 55
Linguistic context 21
Linguistic marker 94
Linguistic modules 54
Linguistics 18
Local focus 120

Macrostructure 44
Multiple access 63
Multiple constraint satisfaction 105
Multi-stage model (of anaphoric
  processing) 105

Necessary inferences 81
Naming task 59
Noun phrase anaphors 100

On-line processing 57

PARSIFAL 76
Performance 18
Phonological component 32
Pragmatic 21
Pragmatically plausible interpretations
  117
Predictive inferences 83
Prime 59
Primitive actions 26
Pro-anaphors 99
Probe 59
Pronouns 93, 99
Pro-sentence 100
Pro-verbs 100
Psycholinguistics 32

Index of Concepts

Register 76
Resolution 97
Resolution processor 97
Rewrite rules 29

SAM (Script Applier Mechanism) 82
Scripts 42
Script Applier Mechanism (SAM) 82
Selection restrictions 35
Semantic features 25
Semantic priming 59
Semantic primitives 26
Semantics 20, 34
Semantics component 32
Sentence representations 34–5
Sentential focus 121
SHRDLU computer program 78
Single stage model (of anaphoric
    processing) 105
Situational context 21

Social context 21
Sociolinguists 18
Speech acts 21
Story gestalts 84
Story grammar 40
Surface structure 31
Synonym 24
Syntactic parser 73
Syntactic priming experiment 71
Syntactic structures 29
Syntax 19
Syntax component 31–2

Target word 59
Time-course 107
Top-down processing 56
Transformational rules 30
Transition networks 73–4

Verb phrase ellipsis (VPE) 101

DISCARD